NAILS *FOREVER*

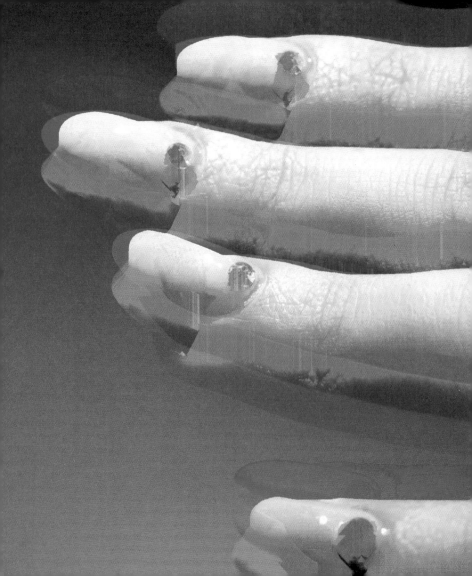

Sharmadean Reid

NAILS *FOREVER*

50 NAIL ART DESIGNS

FROM WAH NAILS LONDON

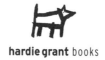

hardie grant books

CONTENTS

NAIL ART TUTORIALS

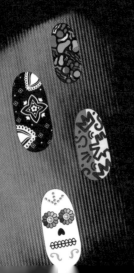

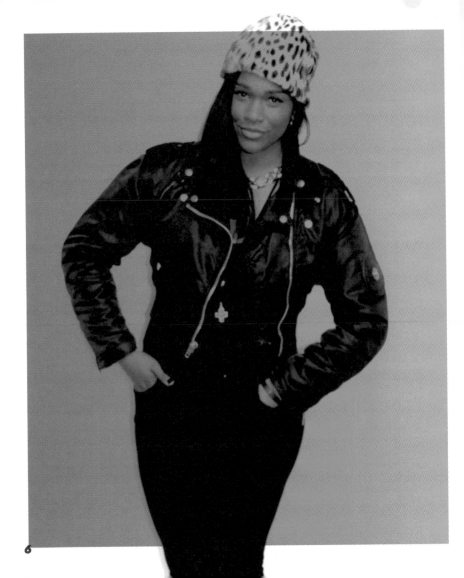

About Wah

In my travels as a stylist, I'd regularly go to Marie Nails in LA and Valley NYC in New York, and I was perplexed as to why London didn't have a cool nail salon of its own, when it's supposed to be a trendsetting city! Then, in 2008, after another bad experience at a hood salon (I wanted a Dior-esque double French, the technician didn't know what Dior was) I got home and told my boyfriend: "You know what? I'm gonna open-up my own nail salon!"

As I spoke the words, the ideas started flowing ... it wasn't just going to be any salon, it was going to be a community for all the local girls in my neighbourhood, and beyond. I wanted to reflect the spirit behind WAH, the girls' fanzine I was making at the time. I had started the blog for the fanzine in 2006 and had gathered an international gang of girls who would crash at each other's houses when they were in town. It was only natural that the salon be called WAH Nails – a physical home for the online community I'd created.

It took a lot of planning and hard work, but after finding a location two minutes from my house in east London, we opened the doors to WAH Nails Dalston in July 2009. I lived in a big loft space at the time, and my friends were always inviting themselves over – fashion designers, DJs, writers, artists – so I knew I had the perfect creative clientele. Soon, the salon became a local hub for different happenings; we hosted Uffie's album party, had exhibitions by local female artists, and held a huge fundraiser for the victims of the Japanese tsunami, with all of our friends donating goods. Sometimes we would all just sit around after hours watching *Paris Is Burning* or Beyonce's tour DVD.

Within a few months we had been featured in *Vogue*, *Elle*, the *New York Times*, *i-D Magazine* ... pretty much every publication worth noting. The fashion press seemed to love it! By November, Selfridges had asked us to host a pop-up salon and we continued to do pop up nail salons across the world. It was a crazy whirlwind but I had achieved what I set out to do.

WAH Nails helped change the culture of nail design. Before we opened, "nail art" was a dirty word within beauty circles, something a bit tacky and ghetto – but I knew it could be more. Nail artists like Marian Newman and Jenny Longworth had been pioneering fashion-forward nail art in magazines for a while, but no one was bringing it to the mainstream. And that's where we came in. Our nail style has now been imitated globally, and our concept – from doing nails in clubs and festivals, to the way we relate to our customers – has infiltrated the nail world ... but there is so much more we still want to do!

Now we have our own product range of nail polishes and nail-art pens called WAH London, and a brand new home in our old stomping ground of Dalston, at 494 Kingsland Road.

The next step is this book, and it's what WAH is all about: sharing our passion, our style, and our technique with you – because everyone deserves hot nails.

Sharmadean Reid
Founder

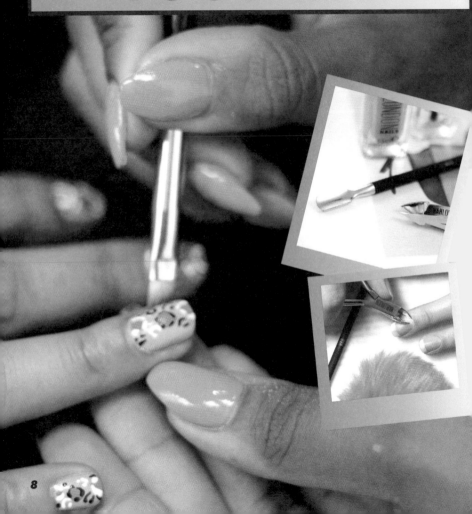

TOOL KIT

Depending on how professional you want to get, your nail kit can be as little as a few polishes, pens and stripers, to a huge case packed with all kinds of nail equipment and goodies! This list covers most of the things that you need to do the designs in this book, although not all are essential. You can do a lot with one polish colour and one nail-art pen. The thing we absolutely recommend is a good topcoat, try our Classy Glassy Glossy! After all your hard work on your nail art, you dont want it ruined by a cheap gloss. If there is one bit of your kit that you spend money on, make sure this is it as a good topcoat will give any cheap polish a smooth, glassy finish.

Trawl the internet, eBay and craft shops for small, fun things to stick on your nails. As long as they are small and flat, it will work. If it's too flat, for example, a metal loveheart, try curving it with pliers so it fits around your nails. If you want a truly personal design, you can also make your own nail art accessories with 3D acrylic and decals!

01 - HAND SANITIZER
Ensure you use hand sanitiser before starting work, in case of any nasty cuts. A non-alcohol based gel or spray will stop your hands drying out.

02 - NAIL FILE
The higher the grit number, the smoother it will be. Get a good quality one that you can wash and reuse.

03 - BLOCK BUFFER
Important for smoothing over the nail but also creating an ideal surface for your polish to stick to.

04 - SHINE BUFFER
If you're going to have your natural base exposed in your design, shine it up!

05 - CUTICLE PUSHER
For lifting the cuticle on the nail plate.

06 - CUTICLE NIPPER
Using them sparingly to cut your cuticles after you've lifted. Beware of cutting your live skin, which frames your nail.

07 - BASE COAT
To help your nail polish stick and protect your nails from staining.

08 - NAIL POLISH COLOURS
You should know what these are by now... Check our WAH London range!

09 - TOP COAT
Totally important for sealing your nail art and adding that glossy finish!

10 - CUTICLE OIL
Essential for combating dryness around the nail that you get from polish remover and keeping your nail bed nourished.

11 - NAIL POLISH REMOVER / ACETONE
For cleaning up your nail design and removing your nail polish or old gel and acrylics.

12 - NAIL-ART PEN
Without these we would not exist — there is so much possibility with a nail pen! Start with black then build your colour collection.

13 - NAIL STRIPERS
Use these for straight lines. To keep your bristles neat, snip any loose hairs with small scissors. If the brush starts to bend, bin it!

14 - EMPTY NAIL STRIPER
Keep an empty bottle filled with polish remover and wipe after each use. Dip into your chosen polish when needed.

15 - SPONGE
Make-up ones are ok, but dishwashing sponges with large holes are great for fades.

16 - TWEEZERS
For applying decals and jewels.

17 - DECAL PAPER
Print your own designs with these.

18 - FIMO CANES
Small canes, usually of fruit or animals, can be sliced really thinly and applied to the nail for decoration.

19 - NAIL WHEEL
Practice your designs on blank nail wheels.

20 - CLEAN-UP BRUSH
For cleaning around your nail if you make a mess. Make sure bristles are short and don't rot in the polish remover.

21 - NAIL JEWELLERY
Great for blinging up your nail. Curve it with pliers for a longer lasting finish.

22 - SWAROVSKI CRYSTALS
Cheap rhinestones don't cut it in our book. If you want proper bling go for crystals!

23 - ORANGE STICK/COCKTAIL STICK
Great for creating swirls and marbling but also for picking up nail studs and jewels.

24 - HAND MOISTURISER
The more you do nails, the drier your hands get from the constant chemical exposure. Keep your hands moisturised!

25 - NAIL GLUE
Use small amounts to stick on any heavy nail accesories.

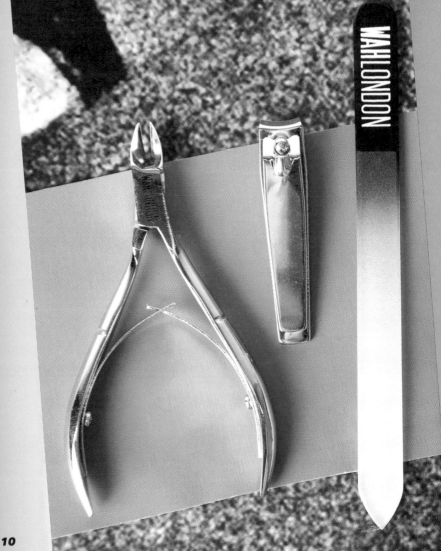

WAHLONDON

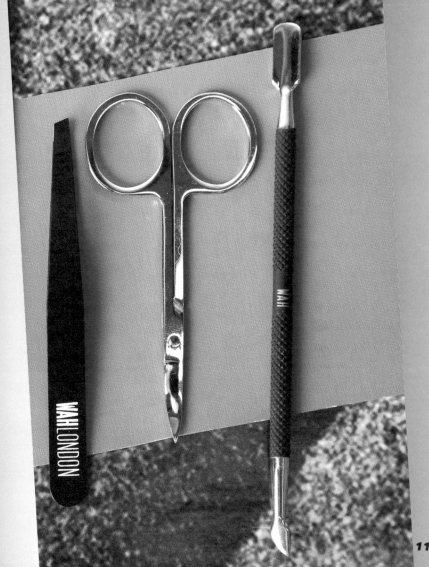

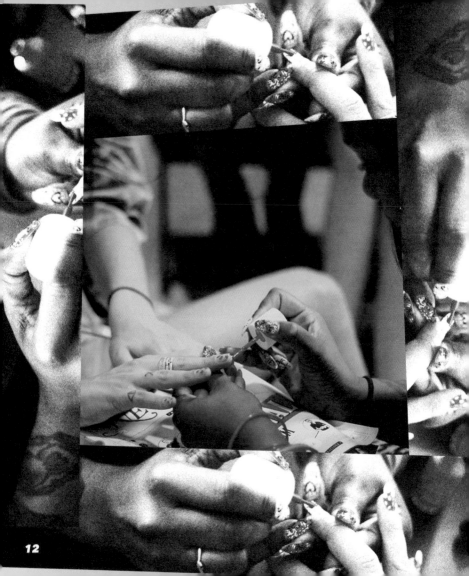

PREP & FINISH

PREPPING YOUR NAILS PROPERLY ENSURES THAT YOUR NAIL POLISH STAYS ON FOR AS LONG AS POSSIBLE! FOLLOW THESE STEPS FOR A PROFESSIONAL FINISH.

PREP

STEP 1 – Before you begin painting, it's crucial to prepare a clean base. Take a lint-free nail wipe and soak it in nail polish remover. Place it over your nail for a few seconds and then pinch in from the sides and sweep down the nail.

STEP 2 – File your nails to the shape you want. Even if you've filed them recently, you may have knocked your nails and caused uneven tips. File using smooth, long motions towards the centre of the nail, from the sides in. Don't file furiously backwards and forwards like you're using a saw because you'll damage your nails. Make sure they're all the same length.

STEP 3 – Using a buffer, buff your nails lightly to create a smooth nail bed. Buffing will also get rid of any ridges. Only buff once a week.

STEP 4 – It's important to dehydrate the nail before you apply the base coat – this will really make the polish stick. Use a lint-free nail wipe soaked in nail polish remover to get rid of any excess oil moisture or dust from buffing. Don't touch your nail bed as the moisture from your fingertips will prevent polish from staying on.

STEP 5 – Now you're ready to use your base coat! Apply a thin layer of base coat to each nail and leave to dry for one to two minutes. All that's left to do now is to choose your nail design!

FINISH

STEP 1 - Once you've finished your nail art or design, wait for five minutes to apply your top coat so you don't smudge your work! Try our WAH London "Classy Glassy Glossy" and apply a generous layer to the nails. Make sure your brush isn't overloaded with polish – you can remove any excess by wiping it across the neck of the polish bottle.

STEP 2 - To perfect your work, always have your clean-up brush ready to get rid of any imperfections. Dip your brush in acetone or nail polish remover and sweep around the cuticle area for a really neat line of polish around the base of your finger.

STEP 3 - To get rid of dry cuticles, apply a swipe of cuticle oil around them. This hydrates the area around the cuticle and leaves a nice, neat, shiny finish.

THERE ARE TWO KEY THINGS YOU NEED TO DO THE NAIL ART IN THIS BOOK: A NAIL-ART PEN AND NAIL ART STRIPER, BOTH WIDELY AVAILABLE ONLINE OR AT YOUR LOCAL NAIL SUPPLY STORE. EXPERIMENT WITH DIFFERENT SIZES AND BRANDS TO FIND WHAT WORKS FOR YOU!

TIPS AND TRICKS

NAIL-ART PENS ARE PENS FILLED WITH NAIL VARNISH THAT YOU SQUEEZE OUT OF A TINY NIB TO DRAW SHAPES AND PATTERNS ON YOUR NAIL.

IT ALSO CONTAIN STRIPERS INSIDE IF YOU SCREW OFF THE NIB!

YOUR NAIL-ART PEN IS YOUR ULTIMATE TOOL SO LOOK AFTER IT. WIPE THE NIB AFTER EACH USE TO ENSURE IT DOESN'T GET BLOCKED.

IF IT DOES GET BLOCKED, SIT THE NIB IN THE TINIEST POOL OF POLISH REMOVER FOR A FEW HOURS TO LET IT DISINTEGRATE THE BLOCKAGE.

IF IT RUNS OUT YOU CAN REFILL IT BY SCREWING OFF THE NIB AND POURING FRESH POLISH OF THE SAME COLOUR INSIDE YOUR PEN.

SQUEEZE YOUR NAIL PEN OUT A TINY BIT ON A SURFACE JUST BEFORE YOU START PAINTING. THIS IS TO GET RID OF ANY AIR BUBBLES, OTHERWISE YOU MAY SPLAT A LOAD OF VARNISH ON YOUR PRISTINE NAIL. SOME OF THE GIRLS IN THE SALON USE THEIR HAND!

14

FOR TINY DOTS AND DETAILED WORK, DON'T SQUEEZE THE PEN ACTUALLY ON THE NAIL. INSTEAD, LET A TINY BALL OF POLISH FORM ON YOUR NIB AND THEN STROKE IT ON THE NAIL IN YOUR DESIRED SHAPE. THIS PREVENTS LARGE BLOBS OF POLISH RUINING YOUR DESIGN.

PRACTISE, PRACTISE, PRACTISE! CONTROLLING YOUR NAIL-ART PEN MAY SEEM TOUGH AT FIRST BUT EVERYONE GETS BETTER WITH PRACTISE.

KEEP YOUR NAIL PENS COOL! WHEN THEY HEAT UP THE VARNISH INSIDE EXPANDS AND FLOWS OUT OF THE NIB TOO QUICKLY, MAKING IT DIFFICULT TO CONTROL. TRY KEEPING THEM IN THE FRIDGE ON A HOT DAY.

YOUR POLISH STRIPER CAN BE A LITTLE MORE UNRULY. BEFORE YOU BUY IT OPEN THE CAP AND CHECK THAT THE BRISTLES ARE POKER STRAIGHT. LIMP BRISTLES ARE UNUSABLE.

WE RECOMMEND ALSO BUYING AN EMPTY STRIPER BOTTLE. FILL IT WITH VARNISH REMOVER AND THEN YOU CAN DIP IT IN ANY NAIL VARNISH COLOUR TO COMPLETE YOUR DESIGN. AFTER USING IT WITH A NEW COLOUR, WIPE THE BRISTLES WITH A LINT-FREE PAD SOAKED IN VARNISH REMOVER AND THEN DIP IN BACK INTO ITS BOTTLE.

WIPE THE CAP AFTER YOUR STRIPER WITH EACH USE – YOU SHOULD BE DOING THIS WITH ALL YOUR NAIL VARNISHES ANYWAY! A CRUSTY CAP ALLOWS AIR TO GET TO THE POLISH WHICH MAKES IT THICKER AND EVENTUALLY UNUSABLE.

WHEN PAINTING STRAIGHT LINES, WIPE ANY EXCESS VARNISH INTO THE LID OF YOUR STRIPER AND THEN INSTEAD OF USING THE TIP TO DRAG THE VARNISH ALONG THE NAIL, LAY THE BRUSH ON THE NAIL AT A FLATTER ANGLE SO YOU ALREADY HAVE HALF OF YOUR LINE DRAWN. THEN COMPLETE BY DRAGGING OFF THE NAIL.

IF YOU FIND YOU HAVE ANY LOOSE BRISTLES, WIPE THE BRUSH CLEAN AND THEN SNIP THEM OFF IMMEDIATELY. THEY CAN RUIN YOUR PERFECT DESIGN.

KEEP YOUR TOOLS NICE AND CLEAN. NOT ONLY IS THIS GOOD FOR HYGIENE, BUT IT ALSO ENSURES YOUR KIT LASTS A LONG TIME!

A NOTE ON THE FLOATING TECHNIQUE: It's important to wait a while to let your nail art settle before applying the topcoat, otherwise you may end up dragging your design and smudging it. But if you really can't bear to wait, we use the floating technique to apply your topcoat onto semi-wet nail designs. Apply a generous blob of polish over the wettest part of your design. Wait a nanosecond and then using your topcoat polish brush, waft or float the topcoat over the nail rather than dragging it in long stripes. You can also just dot blobs of topcoat over parts of your design and then continue topcoating as usual.

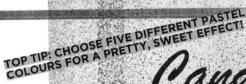

Candystripe

They taste just like candy! Well,
erm, maybe not - but they look just
as sweet!

YOU WILL NEED >
• pink polish
• white nail striper

HOW TO >
Step 1. Paint your nails with the
pink base colour. Allow to dry.

Step 2. Using the white striper,
paint a thin, neat line down the
centre of the nail.

Step 3. Paint a second line, keeping
it to the left of the centre line,
all the way to the tip. Make sure
the lines are evenly spaced.

Step 4. Paint the third line to the
right of the centre line.

Step 5. Continue to work your way
outward, alternating between left
and right, until you reach the edge
of the nail. This will ensure you
get an evenly striped pattern.

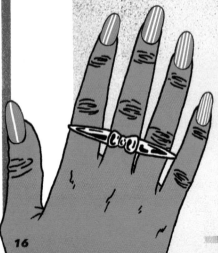

16

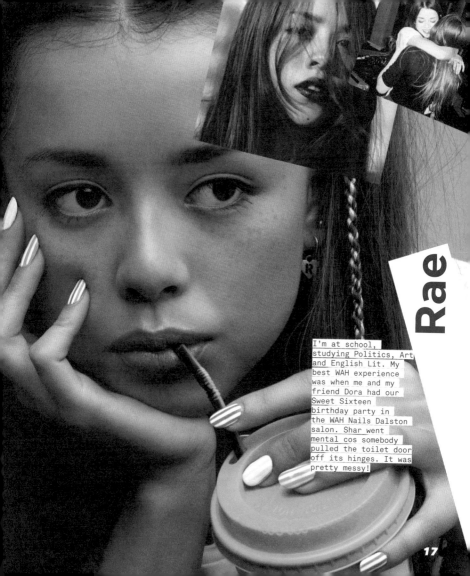

Rae

I'm at school, studying Politics, Art and English Lit. My best WAH experience was when me and my friend Dora had our Sweet Sixteen birthday party in the WAH Nails Dalston salon. Shar went mental cos somebody pulled the toilet door off its hinges. It was pretty messy!

17

Sometimes we joke that a bad leopard print design can often look like bacteria. Then one day we were like, but let's actually do bacteria nails! Our super intern-turned-employee Ellie came up with this design influenced by the incredible art photographer Fabian Oefner, who captures weird scientific phenomena under microscopic lenses and makes it beautiful and pretty. This one can be a little time consuming but the effects are so ridiculously good its defo worth the wait!

YOU WILL NEED
· 7 different coloured neon polishes
· cocktail stick
· black nail-art pen

BACTERIA

STEP 1
Pick your polishes. I recommend neons! Paint a single, thin white base followed by two coats of neon yellow.

STEP 2
Using your choice of polish colours, dab a generous amount onto the nail in spots and blobby shapes. Do this for all of the colours.

STEP 3
While the polish is still wet, use a cocktail stick to swirl and blend the polish together where they meet. This will make new colours.

STEP 5
Top-coat using the floating technique (page 15) so that you don't smear your handiwork.

STEP 4
After this has had a couple of minutes to dry, grab your nail-art pen and outline each colour. Try to keep it very round and almost blob like — mix up your shapes!

TOP TIP
USING A WHITE BASE WILL MAKE YOUR COLOURS POP! DON'T SKIP THIS PART.

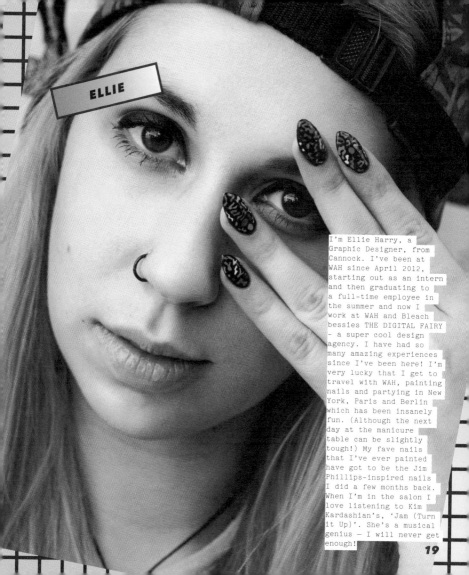

I'm Ellie Harry, a Graphic Designer, from Cannock. I've been at WAH since April 2012, starting out as an intern and then graduating to a full-time employee in the summer and now I work at WAH and Bleach bessies THE DIGITAL FAIRY – a super cool design agency. I have had so many amazing experiences since I've been here! I'm very lucky that I get to travel with WAH, painting nails and partying in New York, Paris and Berlin which has been insanely fun. (Although the next day at the manicure table can be slightly tough!) My fave nails that I've ever painted have got to be the Jim Phillips-inspired nails I did a few months back. When I'm in the salon I love listening to Kim Kardashian's, 'Jam (Turn it Up)'. She's a musical genius – I will never get enough!

19

TOP TIP: CUSTOMIZE THE DESIGN BY USING TWO
OR THREE DIFFERENT COLOURED DOTS, OR EVEN DOING
A THREE-STRIPED BASE WITH LEOPARD PRINT ON TOP!

Leopard

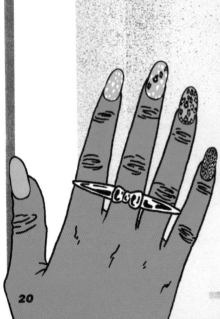

The original WAH girl leopard print
is the design that made our name
famous in the nail world. Sure, we
didn't invent applying leopard print
to nails, but we definitely took it
to the next level. Leopard print is
a classic – it can be grown-up chic
or wild and crazy and can be painted
in so many colourways that you are
guaranteed to find a combination to
suit you.

YOU WILL NEED >
• mint green polish
• white polish
• black nail-art pen

HOW TO >
Step 1. Paint your nails with the
mint green base colour. Allow them
to dry.

Step 2. Take your white nail polish
and, using a semi-dry brush, paint
white strokes dotted around the
nail, starting at the centre.

Step 3. With your black nail-art
pen, make broken circles and semi-
circles around the dots.

Step 4. Continue until all the white
spots are outlined.

Step 5. Fill in the gaps with empty
broken circles and black pen strokes.

20

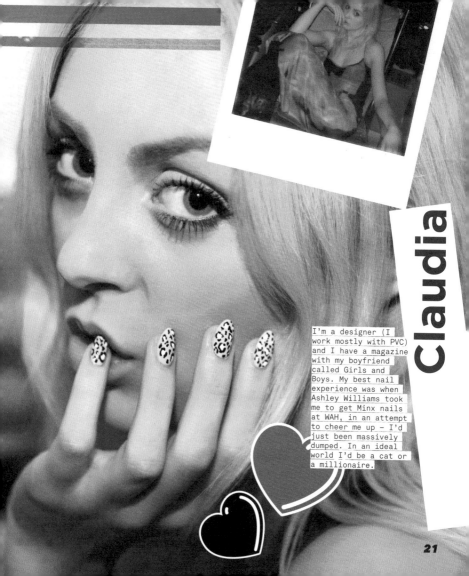

Claudia

I'm a designer (I work mostly with PVC) and I have a magazine with my boyfriend called Girls and Boys. My best nail experience was when Ashley Williams took me to get Minx nails at WAH, in an attempt to cheer me up – I'd just been massively dumped. In an ideal world I'd be a cat or a millionaire.

Every now and then, we all wanna unleash the Chola inside of us and what better way to do this than with some gold hoops, a bit of lip liner and bad-boy bandana nails. These babies take influence from the motifs on our Paisley design (page 72), and with the right colour palette and mix of pattern, you too can make authentic bandana looking nails.

STEP 1
Paint your base colour. Black works really well as does white and other traditional bandana colours. Begin with your teardrop and four-star motifs.

YOU WILL NEED:
· black polish
· white striper
· white nail-art pen

STEP 2
Outline each motif so that they are double ringed.

BANDANA

STEP 5
Add dots on the outline of your teardrops and dots over whole nail as a background print.

STEP 4
Add floral motifs around your four-star.

STEP 3
Paint small diamond shapes in neat rows to form a back pattern.

TOP TIP
TAKE INSPIRATION FROM AN ACTUAL BANDANA AND TRY TO MAKE EACH NAIL UNIQUE, BASED ON A DIFFERENT PART OF THE BANDANA

THE FULL SET!

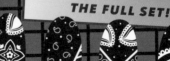

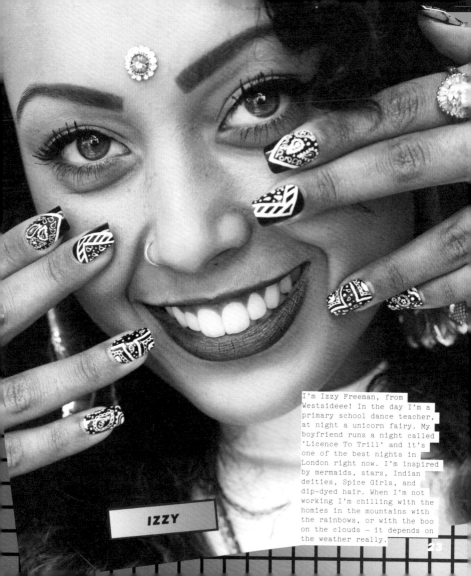

I'm Izzy Freeman, from Westsideee! In the day I'm a primary school dance teacher, at night a unicorn fairy. My boyfriend runs a night called 'Licence To Trill' and it's one of the best nights in London right now. I'm inspired by mermaids, stars, Indian deities, Spice Girls, and dip-dyed hair. When I'm not working I'm chilling with the homies in the mountains with the rainbows, or with the boo on the clouds — it depends on the weather really.

IZZY

23

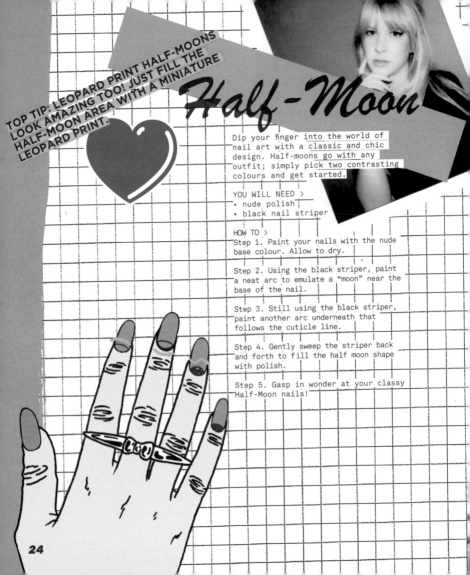

TOP TIP: LEOPARD PRINT HALF-MOONS LOOK AMAZING TOO! JUST FILL THE HALF-MOON AREA WITH A MINIATURE LEOPARD PRINT.

Half-Moon

Dip your finger into the world of nail art with a classic and chic design. Half-moons go with any outfit; simply pick two contrasting colours and get started.

YOU WILL NEED >
• nude polish
• black nail striper

HOW TO >
Step 1. Paint your nails with the nude base colour. Allow to dry.

Step 2. Using the black striper, paint a neat arc to emulate a "moon" near the base of the nail.

Step 3. Still using the black striper, paint another arc underneath that follows the cuticle line.

Step 4. Gently sweep the striper back and forth to fill the half moon shape with polish.

Step 5. Gasp in wonder at your classy Half-Moon nails!

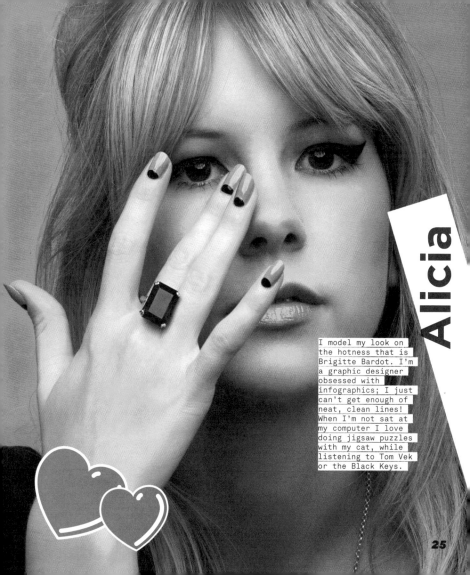

Alicia

I model my look on the hotness that is Brigitte Bardot. I'm a graphic designer obsessed with infographics; I just can't get enough of neat, clean lines! When I'm not sat at my computer I love doing jigsaw puzzles with my cat, while listening to Tom Vek or the Black Keys.

25

This look was inspired by the 90s-style micro-floral dresses we wear all summer, Riot Grrrls, and a general grunge vibe. Black, white and yellow is such a strong colour palette that we knew these nails would work almost immediately. Sometimes the simplest designs are the most beautiful.

GHE20G0TH1K

YOU WILL NEED:
· black polish
· white nail-art pen
· yellow nail-art pen

STEP 1
Paint your base black.

STEP 2
Squeeze your white nail pen gently until a blob of polish has formed on the tip. Make five dots in a circle shape onto the nail. These are your daisy petals.

DAISIES

GHE20G0T

STEP 5
Using your yellow nail pen, squeeze a large yellow dot in the middle of each dotted circle.

STEP 3
Repeat all over the nail until you have four dotted circles.

STEP 4
With your black nail pen, add little flicks in each white petal.

TOP TIP
IF YOU ARE ADEPT WITH YOUR NAIL PEN, YOU CAN FLICK EACH PETAL BLOB INWARDS TO FORM A TEARDROP SHAPE. OTHERWISE A CIRCULAR DOT WILL BE FINE!

26

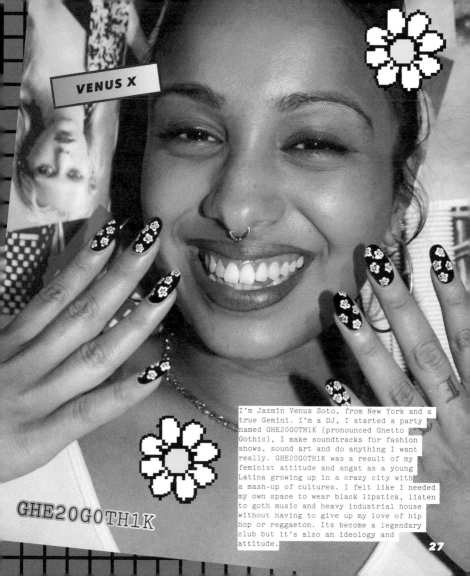

VENUS X

GHE20G0TH1K

I'm Jazmin Venus Soto, from New York and a true Gemini. I'm a DJ, I started a party named GHE20G0TH1K (pronounced Ghetto Gothic), I make soundtracks for fashion shows, sound art and do anything I want really. GHE20G0TH1K was a result of my feminist attitude and angst as a young Latina growing up in a crazy city with a mash-up of cultures. I felt like I needed my own space to wear black lipstick, listen to goth music and heavy industrial house without having to give up my love of hip hop or reggaeton. Its become a legendary club but it's also an ideology and attitude.

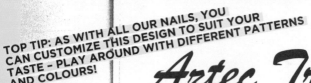
Aztec Tribal

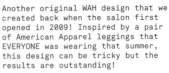

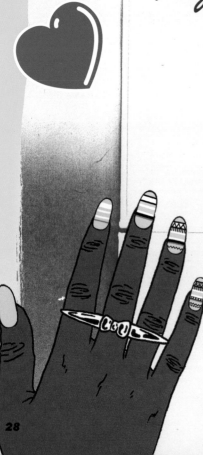

Another original WAH design that we created back when the salon first opened in 2009! Inspired by a pair of American Apparel leggings that EVERYONE was wearing that summer, this design can be tricky but the results are outstanding!

YOU WILL NEED >
• acid green polish
• white nail striper
• pink nail striper
• black nail striper
• black nail-art pen
• white nail-art pen
• LOTS OF PATIENCE!

HOW TO >
Step 1. Paint your nails with the acid green base colour. Allow to dry.

Step 2. Using the white and pink stripers, paint lines across the nail in varying widths, as shown in the illustration.

Step 3. Cement the stripes using the black striper.

Step 4. Take the black nail-art pen and begin adding zig-zag lines and dashes to your design.

Step 5. Add black and white dots where appropriate, or wherever you have room!

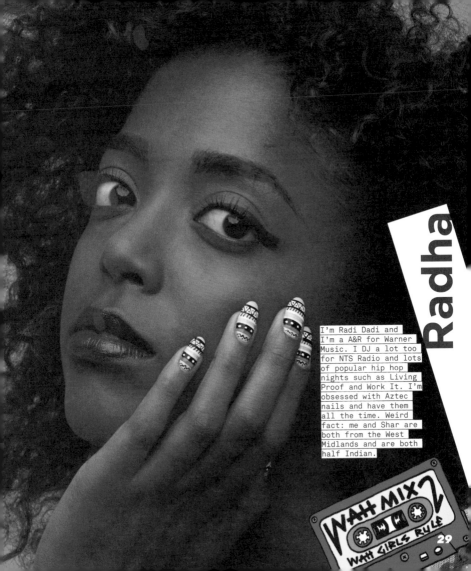

Radha

I'm Radi Dadi and I'm a A&R for Warner Music. I DJ a lot too for NTS Radio and lots of popular hip hop nights such as Living Proof and Work It. I'm obsessed with Aztec nails and have them all the time. Weird fact: me and Shar are both from the West Midlands and are both half Indian.

WAH MIX 2
WAH
WAH GIRLS RULE

The word DOWNTOWN means a lot to us. The majority of WAH Girls are not from the big city, but they have a 'downtown' state of mind. We're all into the same things - art, music, fashion - no matter where we are across the globe, and so we like saying that WAH is for 'Downtown Girls Worldwide'. The downtown nail design here is influenced by the true downtown of New York City, the place that two of our fave artists, Keith Haring and Jean-Michel Basquiat, made their home. Paying homage to their motifs, we've blended the street vibe together to create a fun, pop nail design for the DGW crew.

YOU WILL NEED
· orange polish
· yellow polish
· black nail-art pen

STEP 1
Paint your base nail half orange half yellow. don't worry about doing it neatly as you won't notice any mistakes once you've painted the print.

TOP TIP
CHOOSE THREE OR FOUR LARGE MOTIFS FROM YOUR FAVOURITE ARTISTS AND REPEAT OVER THE NAIL.

DOWNTOWN

STEP 5
Fill in remaining gaps with dots, dashes and commas.

STEP 3
Add dog shapes.

STEP 4
Fill in large gaps with swirls.

STEP 2
Using your black nail-art pen, start with a Basquiat-style crown on each nail. Put them in a different place every time and make some come off the nail.

MOTIF PALETTE

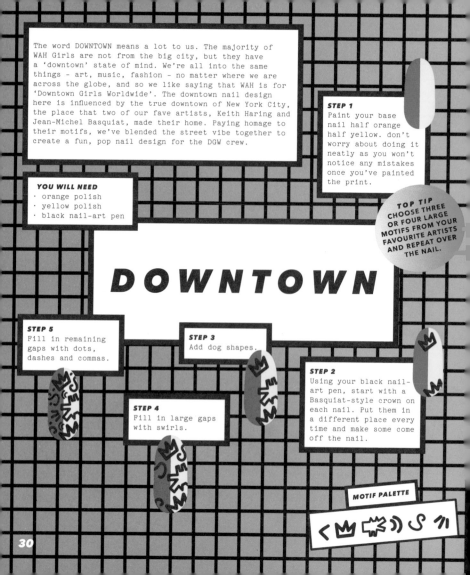

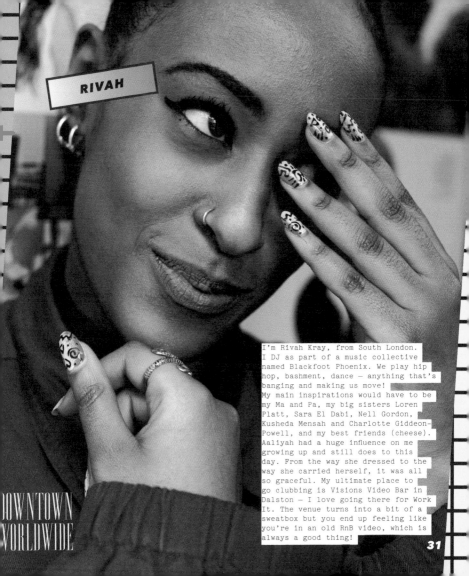

RIVAH

I'm Rivah Kray, from South London.
I DJ as part of a music collective
named Blackfoot Phoenix. We play hip
hop, bashment, dance — anything that's
banging and making us move!
My main inspirations would have to be
my Ma and Pa, my big sisters Loren
Platt, Sara El Dabi, Nell Gordon,
Kusheda Mensah and Charlotte Giddeon-
Powell, and my best friends (cheese).
Aaliyah had a huge influence on me
growing up and still does to this
day. From the way she dressed to the
way she carried herself, it was all
so graceful. My ultimate place to
go clubbing is Visions Video Bar in
Dalston — I love going there for Work
It. The venue turns into a bit of a
sweatbox but you end up feeling like
you're in an old RnB video, which is
always a good thing!

DOWNTOWN
WORLDWIDE

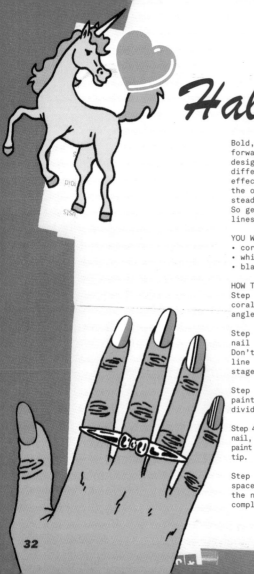

Half-Stripe

Bold, graphic nails for fashion-forward types. The key to this design is painting every nail differently to achieve maximum effect. Although it looks difficult, the only real skill is having a steady hand with your striper brush. So get practising those perfect lines!

YOU WILL NEED >
• coral polish
• white polish
• black nail striper

HOW TO >
Step 1. Paint half the nail with the coral base colour, differing the angle on each finger. Allow to dry.

Step 2. Paint the remainder of the nail with the white base colour. Don't worry about getting a perfect line where the colours meet at this stage. Allow to dry.

Step 3. Using your striper brush, paint a neat, even black line that divides the white from the coral.

Step 4. Working on the white half of the nail, and away from the centre line, paint a second line from the base to the tip.

Step 5. Continue to paint evenly spaced lines towards the edge of the nail until the white section is completely covered in stripes.

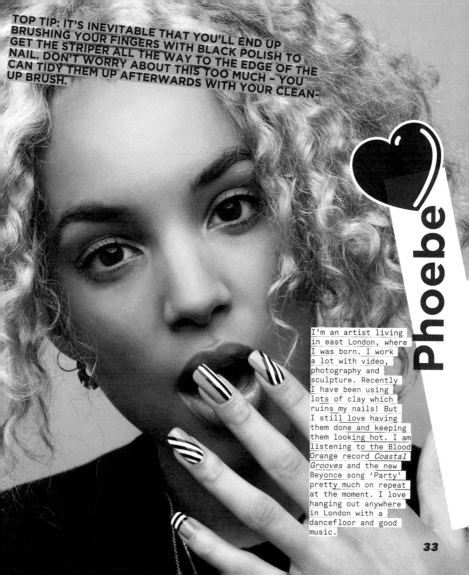

TOP TIP: IT'S INEVITABLE THAT YOU'LL END UP BRUSHING YOUR FINGERS WITH BLACK POLISH TO GET THE STRIPER ALL THE WAY TO THE EDGE OF THE NAIL. DON'T WORRY ABOUT THIS TOO MUCH – YOU CAN TIDY THEM UP AFTERWARDS WITH YOUR CLEAN-UP BRUSH.

Phoebe

I'm an artist living in east London, where I was born. I work a lot with video, photography and sculpture. Recently I have been using lots of clay which ruins my nails! But I still love having them done and keeping them looking hot. I am listening to the Blood Orange record *Coastal Grooves* and the new Beyonce song 'Party' pretty much on repeat at the moment. I love hanging out anywhere in London with a dancefloor and good music.

33

There are so many different types of flower prints out there that you will find endless inspiration if floral nails are your thing. The key with flower prints is highlights. When you've decided on the shade of your flowers, choose a colour from the same family that's lighter and one that's darker. Use all three colours on your flower to add highlights and lowlights for a real print effect. We've gone for a pink rose print with green vines that will give you the basic skills for your own spectacular flower nails.

YOU WILL NEED
· white polish
· dark pink nail striper
· light pink nail striper
· dark green nail-art pen
· light green nail-art pen

FLORAL

STEP 1
Paint your base colour white.

STEP 2
Using your dark pink striper brush, draw a large flower on your nails and two smaller ones coming off the nail.

STEP 3
With the light pink striper, paint a smaller and different flower shape in the gaps.

STEP 4
Using your lighter and darker shades, outline your flowers and the individual petals.

STEP 5
Using two shades of green draw vines and leaves to join your flowers together.

TAKE IT TO THE NEXT LEVEL USE A PAINT PALETTE TO MIX YOUR FLORAL COLOURS TO GIVE YOUR DESIGNS HIGHLIGHT

34

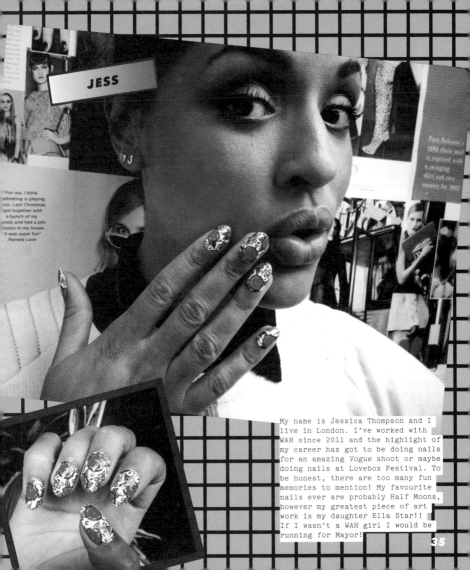

JESS

"For me, I think
celebrating is playing
music. Last Christmas
I got together with
a bunch of my
friends and had a jam
session in my house.
It was super fun"
Pamela Love

My name is Jessica Thompson and I
live in London. I've worked with
WAH since 2011 and the highlight of
my career has got to be doing nails
for an amazing *Vogue* shoot or maybe
doing nails at Lovebox Festival. To
be honest, there are too many fun
memories to mention! My favourite
nails ever are probably Half Moons,
however my greatest piece of art
work is my daughter Ella Star!!
If I wasn't a WAH girl I would be
running for Mayor!

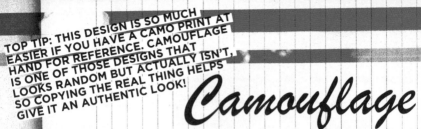
Camouflage

The camo design was inspired by one
of our favourite Japanese streetwear
brands, A Bathing Ape, which is
famous for its camouflage prints.
This looks great with three shades of
the same colour or three completely
contrasting colours, as we've done
here.

YOU WILL NEED >
• neon yellow polish
• pink nail-art pen or polish
• blue nail-art pen or polish

HOW TO >
Step 1. Paint your nails with the
neon yellow base colour. Allow them
to dry.

Step 2. Using your pink nail-art pen
or pink nail polish brush, add some
rounded shapes, like the ones in the
illustration, at the edges of the
nail. Make sure some come right off
the sides of the nail so it looks
like an authentic print.

Step 3. Fill in the centre with more
organic shapes, being careful not to
crowd the nail.

Step 4. Using your blue nail-art pen
or blue polish, paint more circular
shapes and blobs that slightly
overlap the edges of the pink shapes.

Step 5. Check there are no huge gaps,
while ensuring you leave enough room
to keep the base colour visible.

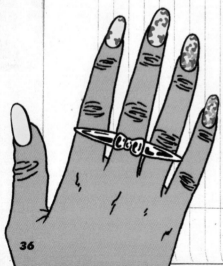

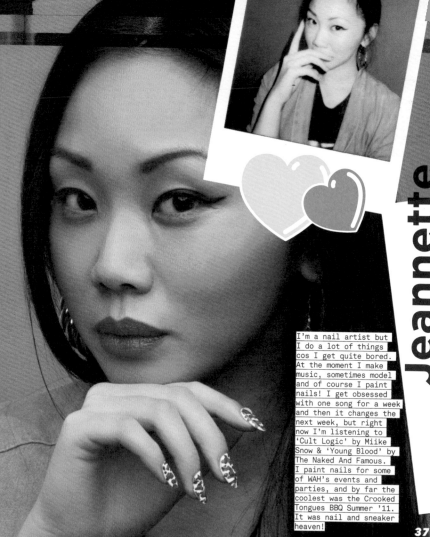

Jeannette

I'm a nail artist but I do a lot of things cos I get quite bored. At the moment I make music, sometimes model and of course I paint nails! I get obsessed with one song for a week and then it changes the next week, but right now I'm listening to 'Cult Logic' by Miike Snow & 'Young Blood' by The Naked And Famous. I paint nails for some of WAH's events and parties, and by far the coolest was the Crooked Tongues BBQ Summer '11. It was nail and sneaker heaven!

37

Galaxy nails are such a fun project! Using a mix of colours and a sponge, treat your nails like a palette mixer. Don't worry about using fresh sponges for each nail — you'll soon get an amazing mix of colours that will add to your design. The white base make the colours pop but if you want a more subtle Galaxy design you can omit this step. Try them! These nails are outta this world! (Sorry, we had to say it…)

YOU WILL NEED

· black polish
· white polish
· paper towel
· a sponge
· magenta pink polish
· light blue polish
· jade green polish
· lilac polish
· purple polish
· orange polish
· yellow polish
· a white nail striper
· a white nail-art pen

GALAXY

STEP 1
Paint your nails with the black base colour and allow it to dry.

STEP 2
Paint white polish on your sponge. Dab the excess off on a paper towel and then lightly dab the sponge on the area you want to create the galaxy appearance on your nail. Go across each nail in different directions.

STEP 5
Use your white nail-art pen to create dots in the black areas to look like stars.

STEP 3
Sponge on two colours per nail onto the white areas you have made. Make sure you overlap them with each other a little.

STEP 4
With a striper create the cross shape over the sponged colours.

TOP TIP
TINY SWAROVSKI CRYSTALS COULD REPLACE THE TINY STARS FOR INTERGALACTIC SPARKLE!

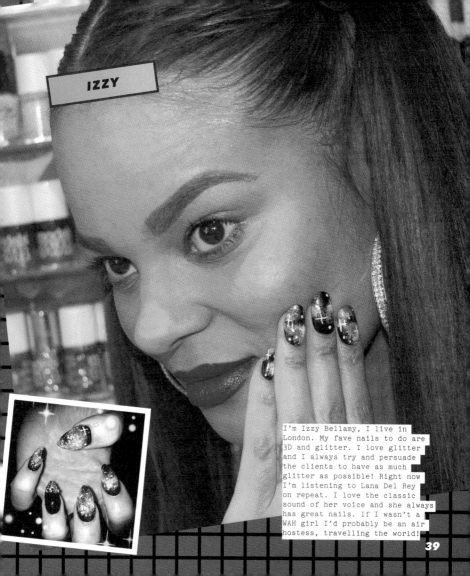

I'm Izzy Bellamy, I live in London. My fave nails to do are 3D and glitter. I love glitter and I always try and persuade the clients to have as much glitter as possible! Right now I'm listening to Lana Del Rey on repeat. I love the classic sound of her voice and she always has great nails. If I wasn't a WAH girl I'd probably be an air hostess, travelling the world!

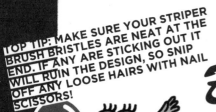

Basketcase

Zoom in on a basket weave for an abstract graphic print.

YOU WILL NEED >
• blue polish
• black nail striper

HOW TO >
Step 1. Paint your nails with the blue base colour. Allow to dry.

Step 2. Using the black striper brush, start at the base of the nail and paint a slightly diagonal line from the left to the right side. Maintain the same pressure on the brush from start to finish to ensure the line looks even. Lift the brush completely off the nail at the end of the line for a clean finish.

Step 3. Repeat above the first line to produce three evenly spaced stripes in black.

Step 4. Working from the tip of the nail, create three more lines, this time at a right angle to the first set.

Step 5. Finish by painting three more lines to create a triangular, woven effect!

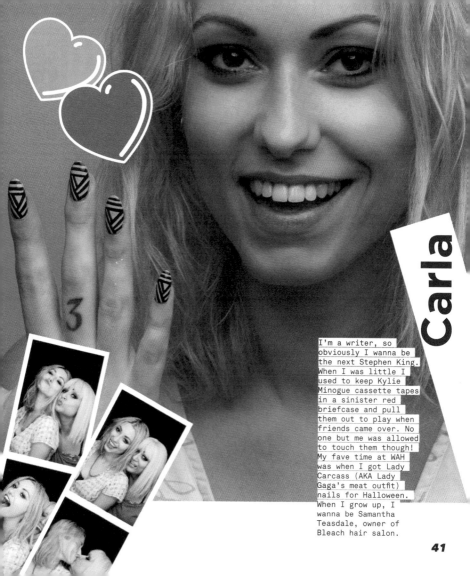

Carla

I'm a writer, so obviously I wanna be the next Stephen King. When I was little I used to keep Kylie Minogue cassette tapes in a sinister red briefcase and pull them out to play when friends came over. No one but me was allowed to touch them though! My fave time at WAH was when I got Lady Carcass (AKA Lady Gaga's meat outfit) nails for Halloween. When I grow up, I wanna be Samantha Teasdale, owner of Bleach hair salon.

41

Okay, I know what you're thinking; this ones gonna take aaaaaages! But no, seriously, we wouldn't do that to you. That's why we are here — to unleash the nail secrets! Houndstooth is such an incred design. The graphic of the monochrome looks amazing on almost any skin tone, or if you're feeling adventurous, try a coloured base.

STEP 2
Paint a thick line (double the width of your striper brush), down the centre of the nails with your striper. Repeat on either side so you have three thick vertical lines.

STEP 3
Repeat but horizontally. One line going across the centre and the then another above and below it.

YOU WILL NEED
· black polish
· white striper
· black striper

STEP 1
Paint all your nails with the black polish.

HOUNDSTOOTH

STEP 5
On the left and top side of each black square, extend the square up with a small line, and across with a small line. See! That was easy!

STEP 4
You'll now have your checkerboard nails. Using your black striper, draw two little lines extending diagonally from the bottom and right side black squares. Be careful not the touch the square below it.

TOP TIP
JUST USE THE VERY TIP OF YOUR BRUSH TO DO THE DIAGONAL LINES, OR A FLICK OF TH NAIL-ART PEN.

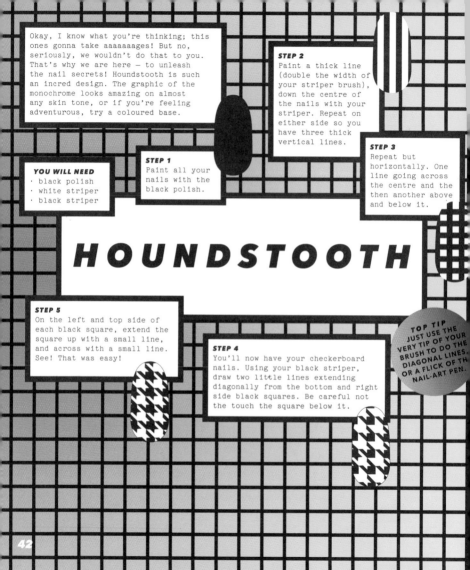

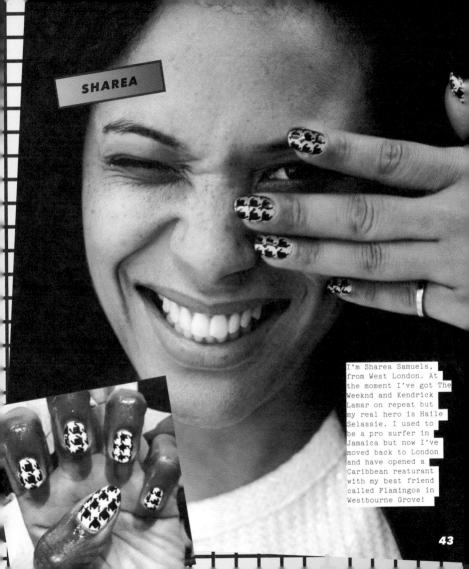

I'm Sharea Samuels, from West London. At the moment I've got The Weeknd and Kendrick Lamar on repeat but my real hero is Haile Selassie. I used to be a pro surfer in Jamaica but now I've moved back to London and have opened a Caribbean reaturant with my best friend called Flamingos in Westbourne Grove!

Letterhead

There's no better way to make a statement than to spell it out on your nails. The first time we did letters for a client – a super-cool graphic designer – she was so specific, she had even printed out the exact font she wanted her boyfriend's name spelled out in! Here we show you a tattoo style... So if you don't want to commit to tattooing LOVE/HATE on your knuckles, write it on your nails instead!

YOU WILL NEED >
• nude polish
• black nail-art pen
• white nail-art pen

HOW TO >
Step 1. Paint your nails with the nude base colour (it looks really effective if you choose one to match your skintone). Allow to dry.

Step 2. Using the black nail-art pen, start to draw the first letter, about 5 mm from the tip of the nail.

Step 3. Work your way down to about 5 mm from the base of the nail, so the letter is centred.

Step 4. When you've finished your letter, add dashes across it for a real Sailor Jerry tat vibe.

Step 5. Highlight certain parts of the letter with white pen, as shown on Gina.

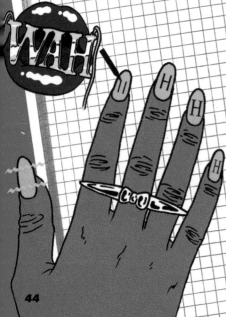

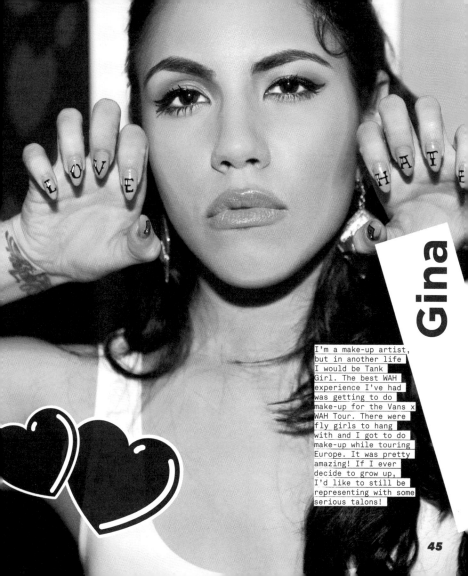

Gina

I'm a make-up artist, but in another life I would be Tank Girl. The best WAH experience I've had was getting to do make-up for the Vans x WAH Tour. There were fly girls to hang with and I got to do make-up while touring Europe. It was pretty amazing! If I ever decide to grow up, I'd like to still be representing with some serious talons!

Japan is our spiritual nail home. If it sparkles, blings, and comes in any shade of pink, it's in! We love doing Japanese-themed nails so much. We wish they'd ship all the fun bits and bobs that you stick on your nails outside of Japan, but unfortunately they don't. So the trick is to hunt online, scour craft stores and bead shops for anything fun that you can stick on your nails. For your own personalised stamp on your nails, you can learn to do 3D acrylic sculptures or create your own 3D shapes using oven-bake clay.

YOU WILL NEED

· 2 different pink glitter polishes
· 1 silver, gold or holographic glitter polish
· Swarovski crystals in a mixture of sizes
· 3D bows and roses
· white nail-art pen

STEP 1

Leave the base of your nail nude. After you've prepped and painted a clear base coat, paint a thin layer of glitter over the top half of your nail, using the first pink glitter.

JAPANESE BLING

STEP 5

Apply topcoat over the whole nail, including all your 3D bits and allow to dry.

STEP 2

Repeat using the second pink glitter and again with your contrast gold or silver glitter.

STEP 3

Using your white nail-art pen draw heart outlines on a few nails.

STEP 4

Using nail glue, stick on crystals, bows and roses. Place most of them on the middle nail doing less on as you go outwards, so the thumb and little finger just have a few crystals on them.

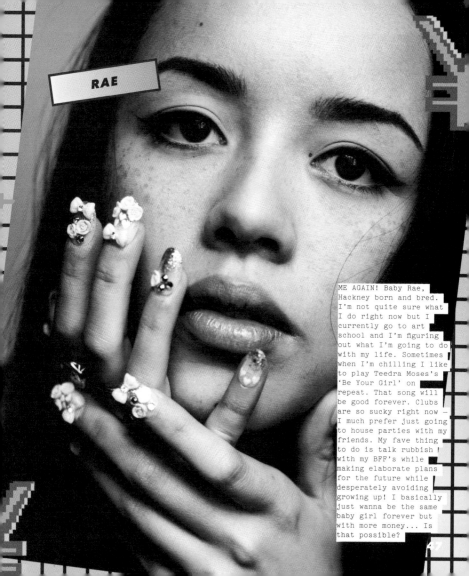

ME AGAIN! Baby Rae, Hackney born and bred. I'm not quite sure what I do right now but I currently go to art school and I'm figuring out what I'm going to do with my life. Sometimes when I'm chilling I like to play Teedra Moses's 'Be Your Girl' on repeat. That song will be good forever. Clubs are so sucky right now — I much prefer just going to house parties with my friends. My fave thing to do is talk rubbish with my BFF's while making elaborate plans for the future while desperately avoiding growing up! I basically just wanna be the same baby girl forever but with more money... Is that possible?

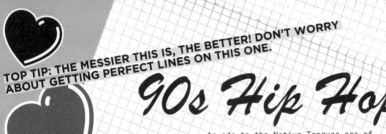

90s Hip Hop

An ode to the Native Tongues era of hip hop, we mix D.A.I.S.Y. Age colours with a distinct ethnic beat.

YOU WILL NEED >
• light purple polish
• yellow polish
• pink polish
• orange polish
• black nail-art pen

HOW TO >
Step 1. Paint your nails with the purple base colour. Allow to dry. Then, using the yellow nail polish, hold your brush at an angle and create short, fat brushstrokes down the centre of the nail in a diamond pattern, as shown in the illustration.

Step 2. Repeat the diamonds using the pink nail polish down the left side of the nail.

Step 3. Do the same with the orange nail polish down the right side of the nail.

Step 4. Gently squeeze the black nail-art pen and apply a thin line to outline all the diamond shapes.

Step 5. Use the pen to add dots inside each diamond and in the empty spaces.

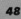

48

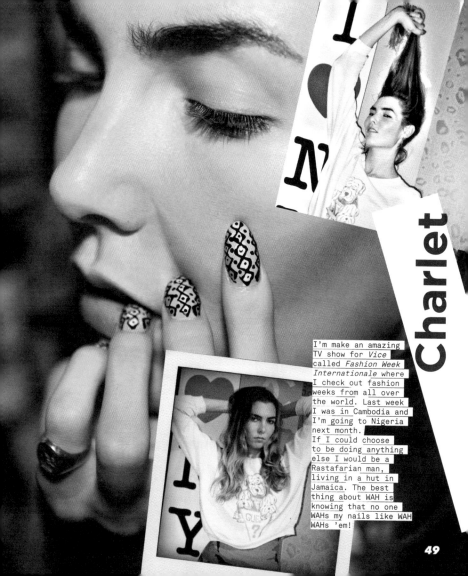

Charlet

I'm make an amazing TV show for *Vice* called *Fashion Week Internationale* where I check out fashion weeks from all over the world. Last week I was in Cambodia and I'm going to Nigeria next month.
If I could choose to be doing anything else I would be a Rastafarian man, living in a hut in Jamaica. The best thing about WAH is knowing that no one WAHs my nails like WAH WAHs 'em!

49

The pointed nail shape, which is so popular right now, lends itself well to this design. Originally starting out as glossy plain hearts on the nail tip, WAH Girl Kat decided to give them a boost with a baby pink base and a super cute doily effect around the heart. This is a great one for Valentine's day!

YOU WILL NEED
· nail file
· pink polish
· red polish
· red striper
· white nail-art pen

LACY HEARTS

STEP 1
File the nail to a pointed tip (this design works best on longer nails). The pointed tip will become the bottom of the heart shape.

STEP 2
Apply a base colour. Pink looks really cute with red but you could try any contrasting colours. Allow to dry.

STEP 3
To create the heart shape, use the red nail polish brush and make a 'V' shape, starting halfway up the nail and brush down to the tip. With a striper dipped into the red polish you can neaten up the shape of the heart. Allow to dry.

STEP 5
Finally, use the white nail-art pen to make some little dots just above the loops which will give a lovely, lacy finish to the heart.

STEP 4
For the lacy effect, take a white nail-art pen and outline the top of the heart. Use the white outline as your guide and make little loops around the top of the heart.

TOP TIP
ENSURE YOUR WHITE NAIL PEN IS COLD. IF IT'S TOO WARM, IT WILL RUN THICK. ALSO DONT SQUEEZE AS YOU ARE PAINTING. SQUEEZE A LITTLE BIT OUT THEN DRAW WITH THE EXCESS.

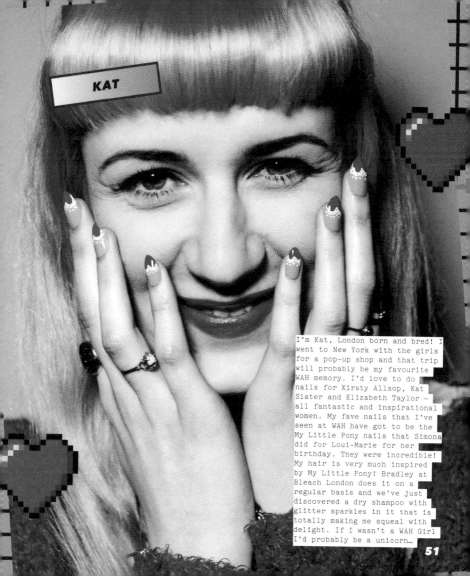

KAT

I'm Kat, London born and bred! I went to New York with the girls for a pop-up shop and that trip will probably be my favourite WAH memory. I'd love to do nails for Kirsty Allsop, Kat Slater and Elizabeth Taylor — all fantastic and inspirational women. My fave nails that I've seen at WAH have got to be the My Little Pony nails that Simona did for Loui-Marie for her birthday. They were incredible! My hair is very much inspired by My Little Pony! Bradley at Bleach London does it on a regular basis and we've just discovered a dry shampoo with glitter sparkles in it that is totally making me squeal with delight. If I wasn't a WAH Girl I'd probably be a unicorn...

TOP TIP: WAIT FOR THE BASE COLOURS TO DRY COMPLETELY BEFORE APPLYING THE WHITE EXPLOSIONS – IF THEY'RE STILL WET, THEY COULD STAIN THE WHITE.

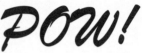

POW!

Because we're all superwomen, we like to wow people with these POW! nails. Inspired by a love of comics and the artist Roy Lichtenstein, we came up with these nails when we first opened the salon – and it's still one of our most popular designs!

YOU WILL NEED >
• five different polishes
• white nail-art pen
• black nail-art pen

HOW TO >
Step 1. Paint each of your nails with a different base colour. Allow to dry.

Step 2. Paint a white 'explosion' in the base corner of each nail using the white nail-art pen.

Step 3. Paint neat polka dots over the top half of the nail.

Step 4. Once each 'explosion' is dry, use your black nail-art pen to write POW! CRASH! BANG! WHAM! and any other comic-book words you want within them.

Step 5. Outline the explosions with your black nail-art pen.

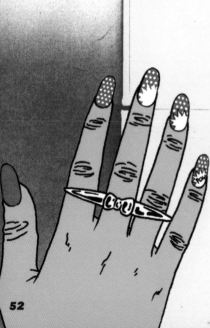

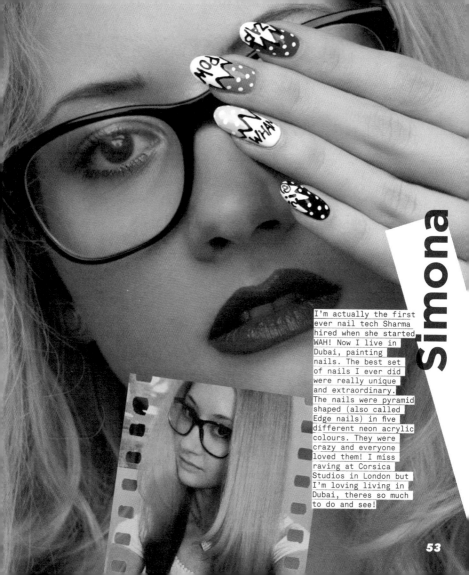

Simona

I'm actually the first ever nail tech Sharma hired when she started WAH! Now I live in Dubai, painting nails. The best set of nails I ever did were really unique and extraordinary. The nails were pyramid shaped (also called Edge nails) in five different neon acrylic colours. They were crazy and everyone loved them! I miss raving at Corsica Studios in London but I'm loving living in Dubai, theres so much to do and see!

A WAH classic, OG design and favourite amongst all our nail techs. The leopard print design is like a finger print, everyone does it differently but one thing's for sure, it always looks FIYAH! Here we show you a basic version with a simple fade underneath so you can updated your technique.

STEP 1
Paint your nails in your base colour — here we've done alternate fingers.

STEP 2
Working on one finger at a time, using your second colour, thickly paint about a third of your nail starting from the tip.

YOU WILL NEED
· yellow polish
· orange polish
· pink polish
· purple polish
· black nail pen
· sponge

LEOPARD FADE

STEP 5
Fill in any gaps with semi circles and commas.

STEP 3
With your sponge, dab the wet polish down the nail to make a fade. Allow it to dry.

STEP 4
Using you nail-art pen, start in the centre of the nail with one broken circle/triangle. Using the first circle as a guide work outwards making the shapes smaller.

TOP TIP
ENSURE YOUR LEOPARD DESIGN GOES OFF THE NAIL FOR A TRUE PRINT EFFECT.

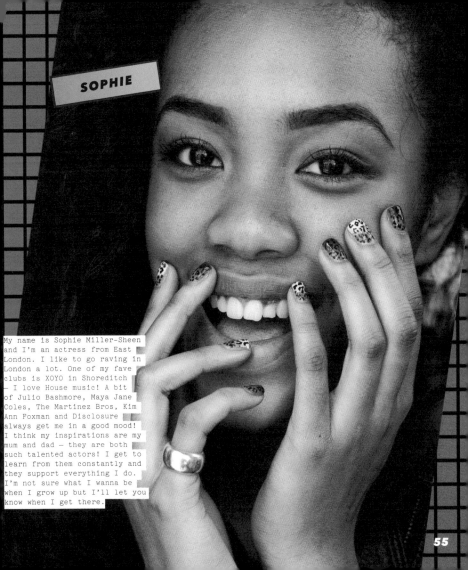

SOPHIE

My name is Sophie Miller-Sheen and I'm an actress from East London. I like to go raving in London a lot. One of my fave clubs is XOYO in Shoreditch — I love House music! A bit of Julio Bashmore, Maya Jane Coles, The Martinez Bros, Kim Ann Foxman and Disclosure always get me in a good mood! I think my inspirations are my mum and dad — they are both such talented actors! I get to learn from them constantly and they support everything I do. I'm not sure what I wanna be when I grow up but I'll let you know when I get there.

TOP TIP: TRY AND PAINT THE WORDS IN DIFFERENT POSITIONS ON EVERY NAIL FOR A COOL PATTERNED EFFECT!

Fash Life

For those on the merry-go-round that is the international fashion-week cycle, this design – a distinctive homage to the legendary artist Stephen Sprouse – should make the madness just a little bit prettier.

YOU WILL NEED >
• yellow polish
• pink polish
• orange polish
• black nail-art pen

HOW TO >
Step 1. Paint alternate nails with the yellow, pink and orange base colours. Allow to dry.

Step 2. Using the black nail-art pen, start at the tip by writing NEW YORK across your nail. Make sure you allow some letters to run off the edge of the nail to give it a real "print" effect.

Step 3. When you get to the edge of the nail, carry the word over to the next line. You will end up breaking words in half – but that's the idea!

Step 4. Continue down the nail, writing from left to right, adding the world's other famous fashion cities – PARIS, LONDON (obvs), TOKYO, MILAN – or whatever cities you want to rep!

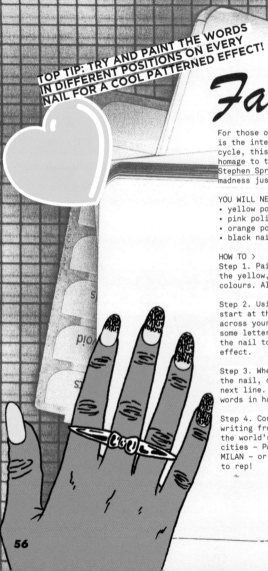

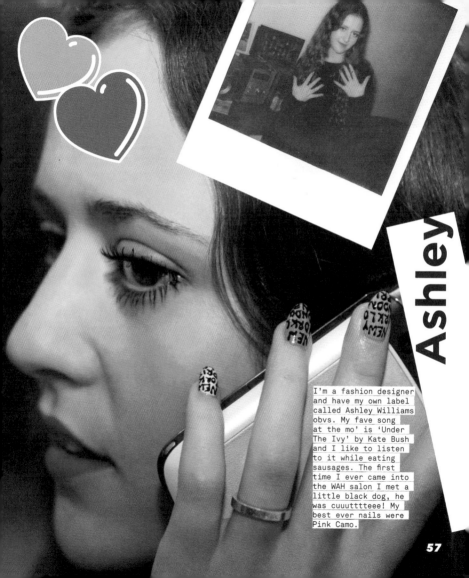

Ashley

I'm a fashion designer and have my own label called Ashley Williams obvs. My fave song at the mo' is 'Under The Ivy' by Kate Bush and I like to listen to it while eating sausages. The first time I ever came into the WAH salon I met a little black dog, he was cuuutttteee! My best ever nails were Pink Camo.

Eye designs are massively popular in the WAH Nails salon, ranging from Turkish evil eyes to gory bloodshot ones. We decided to beautify one of our classics with a Manga-style eye.

YOU WILL NEED

· white striper
· lilac polish
· blue polish
· green polish
· yellow polish
· pink polish
· black nail-art pen
· white nail-art pen
· black striper

MANGA EYES

STEP 1
Paint a couple of coats of your base colour.

STEP 2
Using your white striper, paint outlines of your eyes and fill them in. Keep them big and Manga-like!

STEP 3
Pick three polishes from the same colour palette and, using a clean striper, paint the iris of the eye using one of them. Use the other two polishes to add flecks in the iris — magical!

STEP 4
Pick up your black pen and draw the eye's pupil. Allow to dry then using a white nail-art pen add a little star or heart followed by two smaller white dots for cute light reflections.

STEP 5
Lastly, use your black striper to add full on lashes like you wish your mascara did. Don't forget to topcoat!

TOP TIP
DRAW A FEW MANGA EYES OUT IN YOUR SKETCHBOOK TO GET IT JUST RIGHT. DONT FORGET TO ADD THE WHITE DOTS ON THE IRIS! IT'S WHAT MAKES THE EYE LOOK BIG AND CARTOONY!

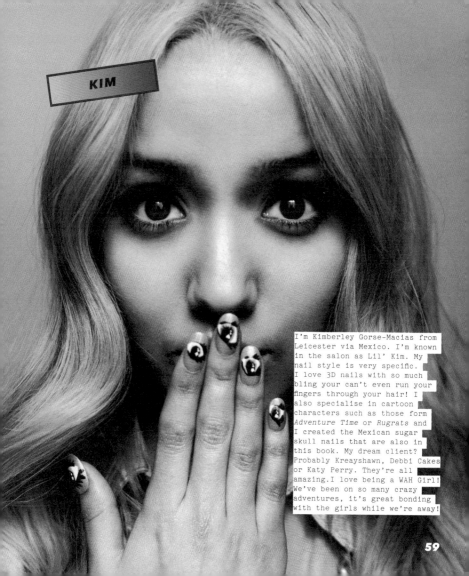

KIM

I'm Kimberley Gorse-Macias from
Leicester via Mexico. I'm known
in the salon as Lil' Kim. My
nail style is very specific.
I love 3D nails with so much
bling your can't even run your
fingers through your hair! I
also specialise in cartoon
characters such as those form
Adventure Time or *Rugrats* and
I created the Mexican sugar
skull nails that are also in
this book. My dream client?
Probably Kreayshawn, Debbi Cakes
or Katy Perry. They're all
amazing.I love being a WAH Girl!
We've been on so many crazy
adventures, it's great bonding
with the girls while we're away!

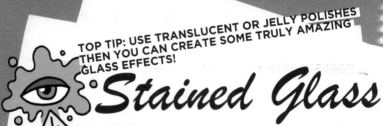

TOP TIP: USE TRANSLUCENT OR JELLY POLISHES THEN YOU CAN CREATE SOME TRULY AMAZING GLASS EFFECTS!

Stained Glass

Go colour crazy by imitating the ancient art of stained glass with these pretty patterned nails.

YOU WILL NEED >
- yellow polish
- blue polish
- pink polish
- lime green polish
- black nail-art pen

HOW TO >
Step 1. Using your yellow nail polish brush, paint three dabs on the nail, spaced far apart. Hold the brush flat so you get a squarish mark.

Step 2. Paint a few blue dabs, close to, but not overlapping, the yellow.

Step 3. Add some pink, being careful not to touch the other colours.

Step 4. Fill in the remaining gaps with the lime green nail polish.

Step 5. Using your black nail-art pen, outline all the colours to create a stained-glass effect.

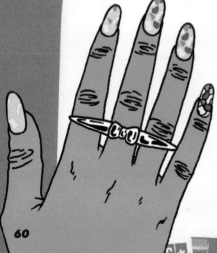

60

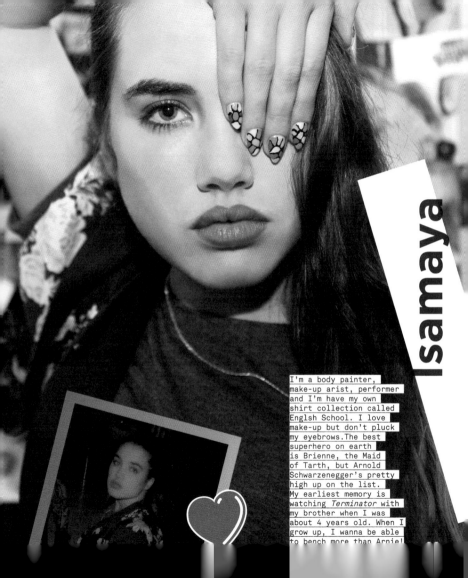

samaya

I'm a body painter, make-up arist, performer and I'm have my own shirt collection called Englsh School. I love make-up but don't pluck my eyebrows. The best superhero on earth is Brienne, the Maid of Tarth, but Arnold Schwarzenegger's pretty high up on the list. My earliest memory is watching *Terminator* with my brother when I was about 4 years old. When I grow up, I wanna be able to bench more than Arnie!

Our little Mexican firecracker, Kim, created these nails and they're pretty much the only requested design on the 'Day of the Dead' festival days. Although intricate, the loops and lacy effects are manageable when you get a rhythm going. Fimo cane flowers can be bought online for a 3D effect but if they're not available you can draw the flowers on instead using a pink nail-art pen.

YOU WILL NEED

· white polish
· black striper
· black nail pen
· flower fimo canes
· top coat
· pink nail-art pen
· blue nail pen
· gold bullion beads
· Swarovski crystals

MEXICAN SKULLS

STEP 1
Apply your white polish as your base colour.

STEP 2
Using a black striper, make the long line to start the teeth. Using the black nail pen create the scallop design along the black line to create the teeth.

STEP 3
With your black striper draw a small upside down heart for the nose. Start by dotting two black dots and dragging the polish to meet in the middle.

STEP 4
Using pre-sliced flower fimos, stick them on with a topcoat to make the eyes, then add two crystals to the centre of the flowers.

STEP 5
Get creative! Using pens, gold beads and crystals to add different motifs of flowers, hearts and dots to decorate your skulls.

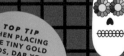

TOP TIP
WHEN PLACING THE TINY GOLD BEADS, DAB YOUR AREA WITH TOPCOAT THEN WORK SUPER FAST PICKING THEM UP WITH A COCKTAIL STICK.

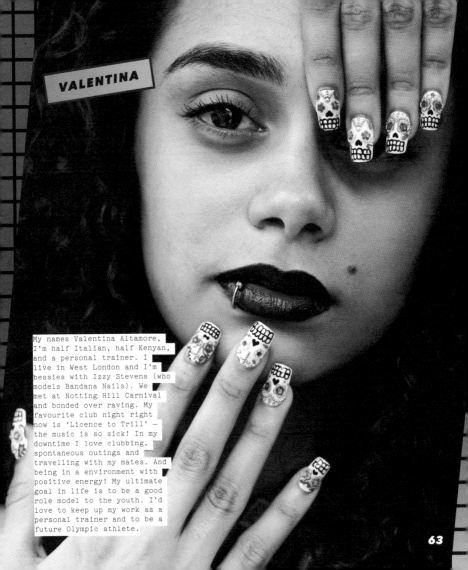

VALENTINA

My names Valentina Altamore,
I'm half Italian, half Kenyan,
and a personal trainer. I
live in West London and I'm
bessies with Izzy Stevens (who
models Bandana Nails). We
met at Notting Hill Carnival
and bonded over raving. My
favourite club night right
now is 'Licence to Trill' —
the music is so sick! In my
downtime I love clubbing,
spontaneous outings and
travelling with my mates. And
being in a environment with
positive energy! My ultimate
goal in life is to be a good
role model to the youth. I'd
love to keep up my work as a
personal trainer and to be a
future Olympic athlete.

Shatter

Shatter-effect polish is one of our fave innovations in nail technology and we love experimenting with different ways to use it! Try this background fade effect for super fashion-forward nails.

YOU WILL NEED >
• blue polish
• yellow polish
• cocktail stick
• black WAH Nails Smash-Up polish

HOW TO >
Step 1. Paint the bottom part of the nail with the blue nail polish, just over the halfway mark. Use quite a lot of polish as you want it to be pretty wet.

Step 2. Paint the top half of the nail with the yellow nail polish, overlapping the blue slightly.

Step 3. While the polish is still wet, use your cocktail stick to blend the colours together on the nail to create a fade effect. Repeat steps 1–3 on each nail individually.

Step 4. Once your nails are completely dry, paint over the colour fade using your Smash-Up polish. Don't worry, you haven't ruined your nails!

Step 5. Watch in wonder and amazement as the polish splits and you get the Smash-Up effect!

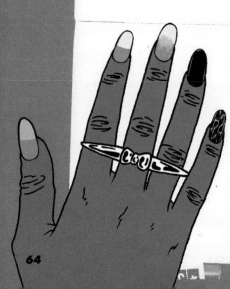

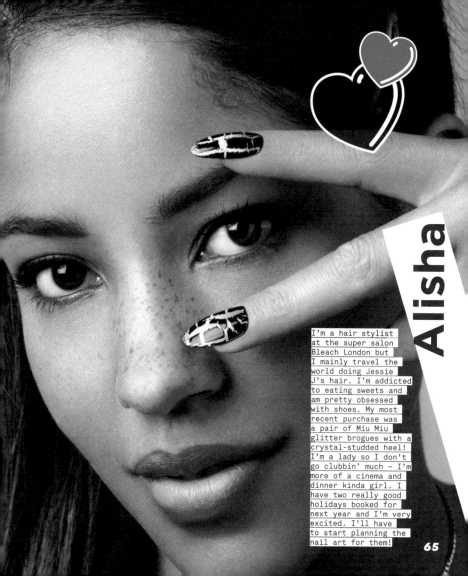

Alisha

I'm a hair stylist at the super salon Bleach London but I mainly travel the world doing Jessie J's hair. I'm addicted to eating sweets and am pretty obsessed with shoes. My most recent purchase was a pair of Miu Miu glitter brogues with a crystal-studded heel! I'm a lady so I don't go clubbin' much – I'm more of a cinema and dinner kinda girl. I have two really good holidays booked for next year and I'm very excited. I'll have to start planning the nail art for them!

65

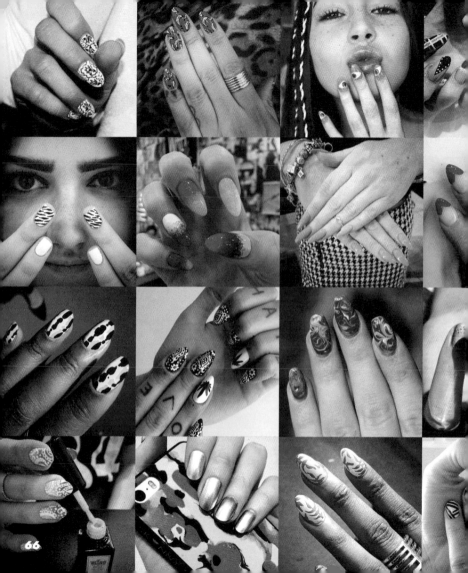

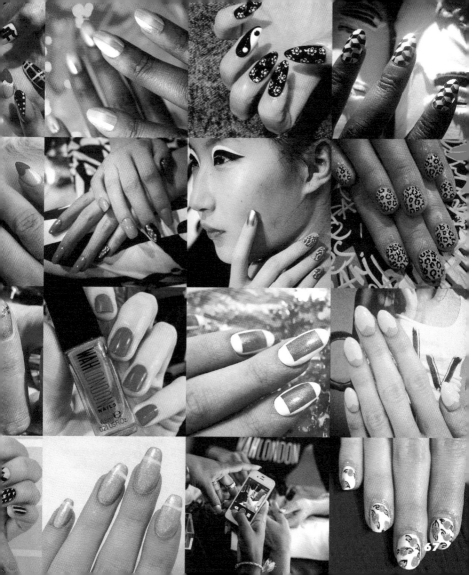

67

We love Pendleton clothing and blankets! The traditional Indian woven fabric patterns lend themselves perfectly to nail designs with their bright colours and bold prints. Choose an ombre of colours of similar shade, but be sure to include a turquoise colour for a true Native American feel.

YOU WILL NEED

· nude polish
. yellow polish
· red polish
· purple polish
· turquoise polish
· black striper

NAVAJO

STEP 1
Paint your base colour nude and allow it to dry. Starting from the middle of the nail, make horizontal lines using your coloured polishes. Work your way through the spectrum of colours so that they mirror each other from the top and bottom of the nail.

STEP 2
For the Native American style designs you will need a black striper. Using the background stripes as a guideline, make little triangle shapes starting from the middle of the nail and working your way out.

STEP 5
Repeat similar, but designs on each nail. Just make sure they're symmetrical.

STEP 4
From the corners of each nail make thin 'V' shapes which frame the nail and black them out with the striper.

STEP 3
Emphasise the triangles by blacking the spaces between each one.

THE FULL SET!

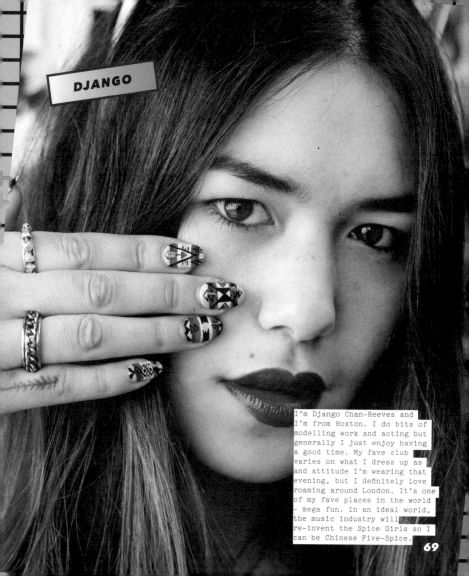

DJANGO

I'm Django Chan-Reeves and I'm from Hoxton. I do bits of modelling work and acting but generally I just enjoy having a good time. My fave club varies on what I dress up as and attitude I'm wearing that evening, but I definitely love roaming around London. It's one of my fave places in the world – mega fun. In an ideal world, the music industry will re-invent the Spice Girls so I can be Chinese Five-Spice.

69

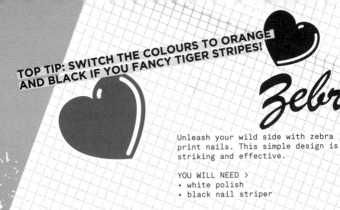

Zebra

Unleash your wild side with zebra print nails. This simple design is striking and effective.

YOU WILL NEED >
• white polish
• black nail striper

HOW TO >
Step 1. Paint your nails with the white base colour. Allow to dry.

Step 2. Using the black striper, start at the base of the nail and paint evenly spaced stripes in black, from the left side of the nail to the centre. To do this, press down heavily on the brush as you begin at the edge of the nail, gradually releasing the pressure as you reach the centre. This will create a triangular-shaped line.

Step 3. Work your way to the tip of the nail to produce three or four evenly spaced stripes.

Step 4. Repeat on the right side of the nail, filling the gaps created by the lines just painted.

Step 5. Gawp at your seriously cute nails!

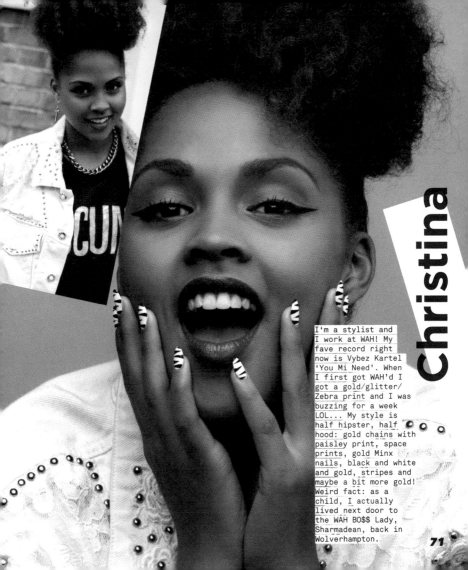

Christina

I'm a stylist and I work at WAH! My fave record right now is Vybez Kartel 'You Mi Need'. When I first got WAH'd I got a gold/glitter/Zebra print and I was buzzing for a week LOL... My style is half hipster, half hood: gold chains with paisley print, space prints, gold Minx nails, black and white and gold, stripes and maybe a bit more gold! Weird fact: as a child, I actually lived next door to the WAH BO$$ Lady, Sharmadean, back in Wolverhampton.

Originating from India via a small town in Scotland, the Paisley design is an intricate but beautiful print on your nails. Take inspiration from the 1970s with a muted colour palette, or go bold with white and blue.

STEP 1
Paint your base colour purple and allow to dry.

STEP 2
Using your nail pen, paint a large teardrop shape in a different place on each nail. Add two smaller teardrop shapes coming off the nail.

YOU WILL NEED
· purple polish
· white nail pen

PAISLEY

STEP 5
Add dots and small commas all over the nail for background effect.

STEP 3
Add a smaller teardrop shape inside the large ones. Some can be solid, some can be outlines.

STEP 4
Outline each teardrop with loops and dots.

TOP TIP
THE POLISH IN WHITE NAIL PENS CAN BE A THICKER TEXTURE. USE A LIGHT BACKGROUND WITH BLACK NAIL PEN IF YOU ARE FINDING YOUR DESIGN IS TOO BLOBBY!

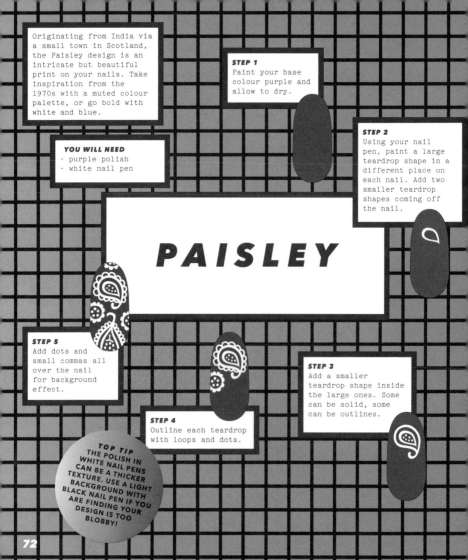

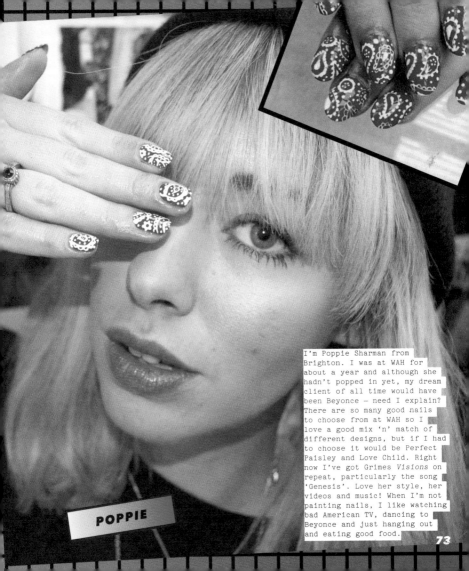

I'm Poppie Sharman from Brighton. I was at WAH for about a year and although she hadn't popped in yet, my dream client of all time would have been Beyonce — need I explain? There are so many good nails to choose from at WAH so I love a good mix 'n' match of different designs, but if I had to choose it would be Perfect Paisley and Love Child. Right now I've got Grimes *Visions* on repeat, particularly the song 'Genesis'. Love her style, her videos and music! When I'm not painting nails, I like watching bad American TV, dancing to Beyonce and just hanging out and eating good food.

POPPIE

Bows

Perfectly pretty fingertips get
wrapped up in bows. Pick light and
girly colours for maximum sweetness.

YOU WILL NEED >
• mint polish
• pink polish
• white nail striper/nail-art pen
• black nail-art pen

HOW TO >
Step 1. Paint your nails alternately
with the mint and pink nail polish.
Allow to dry.

Step 2. With the white striper, paint
a cross near the tip of each nail.

Step 3. Still using the white
striper, paint vertical lines to
connect the cross, to making a bow
shape.

Step 4. Fill in the bow with white polish.

Step 5. Squeeze your white nail-art
pen until a tiny white ball of polish
forms on the end of the nib. Stop
squeezing and gently touch the ball
into the middle of the bow, pushing it
out to create a circle in the centre.

Step 6. Outline the whole bow using
your black nail-art pen. Finish it by
adding two pinch lines off the middle
of each bow.

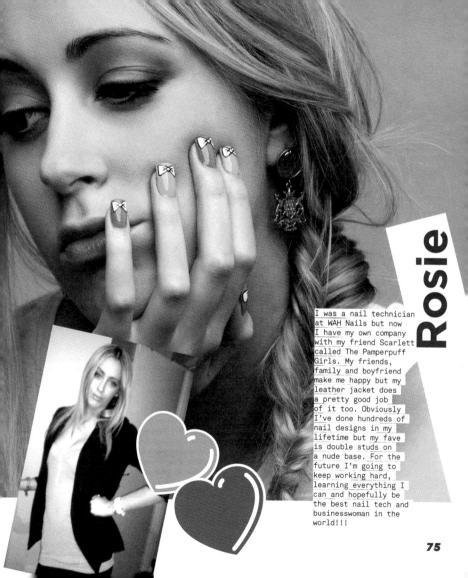

Rosie

I was a nail technician at WAH Nails but now I have my own company with my friend Scarlett called The Pamperpuff Girls. My friends, family and boyfriend make me happy but my leather jacket does a pretty good job of it too. Obviously I've done hundreds of nail designs in my lifetime but my fave is double studs on a nude base. For the future I'm going to keep working hard, learning everything I can and hopefully be the best nail tech and businesswoman in the world!!!

Here at WAH we are all about super island vibes! Everything about the salon is tropical, from the colour palette to our original designs. Grab your rum punch and get tropical with this palm leaf print.

YOU WILL NEED
· neon green polish
· black striper

STEP 1
Paint your base colour neon green.

STEP 2
Using your black striper, draw a diagonal line coming from the bottom right of your nail then gently press the tip of your brush along the line to make small feather-like strokes.

PALM LEAF

STEP 5
Paint two smaller mini leaves coming off the side of the nail.

STEP 3
Paint four more leaves coming off the branch.

STEP 4
Repeat steps 2-3 to create another palm leaf opposite your first one.

TOP TIP IF YOUR STRIPER BRUSH HAS A WAYWARD BRISTLE THIS CAN RUIN YOUR DESIGN. KEEP YOUR STRIPER CLEAN AND SNIP OFF ANY LOOSE BRISTLES WITH NAIL SCISSORS.

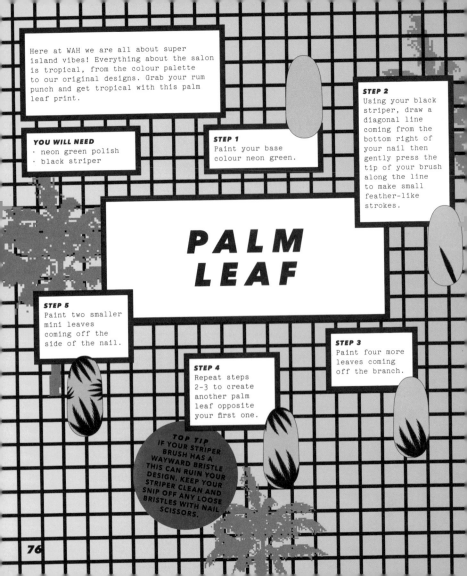

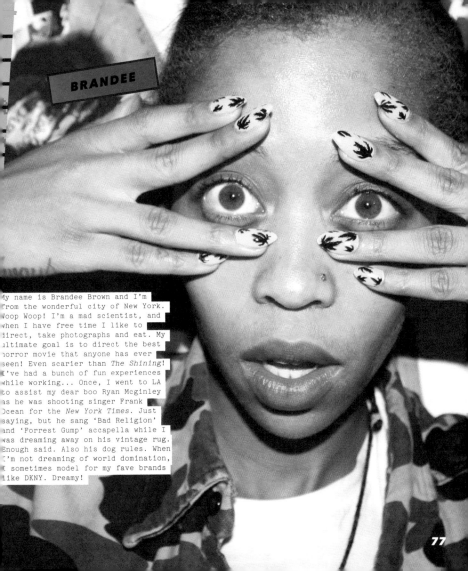

My name is Brandee Brown and I'm from the wonderful city of New York. Woop Woop! I'm a mad scientist, and when I have free time I like to direct, take photographs and eat. My ultimate goal is to direct the best horror movie that anyone has ever seen! Even scarier than *The Shining*! I've had a bunch of fun experiences while working... Once, I went to LA to assist my dear boo Ryan Mcginley as he was shooting singer Frank Ocean for the *New York Times*. Just saying, but he sang 'Bad Religion' and 'Forrest Gump' accapella while I was dreaming away on his vintage rug. Enough said. Also his dog rules. When I'm not dreaming of world domination, I sometimes model for my fave brands like DKNY. Dreamy!

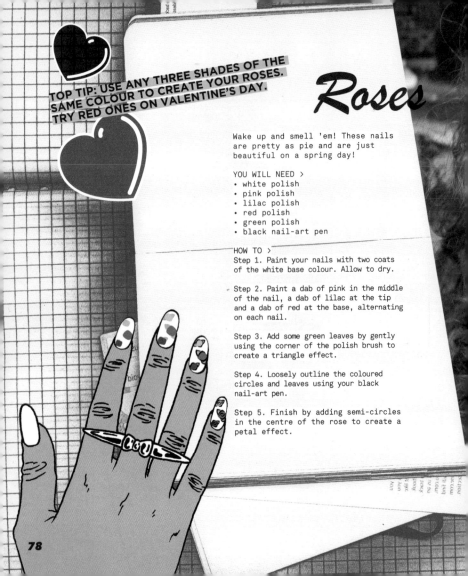

TOP TIP: USE ANY THREE SHADES OF THE
SAME COLOUR TO CREATE YOUR ROSES.
TRY RED ONES ON VALENTINE'S DAY.

Roses

Wake up and smell 'em! These nails
are pretty as pie and are just
beautiful on a spring day!

YOU WILL NEED >
- white polish
- pink polish
- lilac polish
- red polish
- green polish
- black nail-art pen

HOW TO >
Step 1. Paint your nails with two coats
of the white base colour. Allow to dry.

Step 2. Paint a dab of pink in the middle
of the nail, a dab of lilac at the tip
and a dab of red at the base, alternating
on each nail.

Step 3. Add some green leaves by gently
using the corner of the polish brush to
create a triangle effect.

Step 4. Loosely outline the coloured
circles and leaves using your black
nail-art pen.

Step 5. Finish by adding semi-circles
in the centre of the rose to create a
petal effect.

78

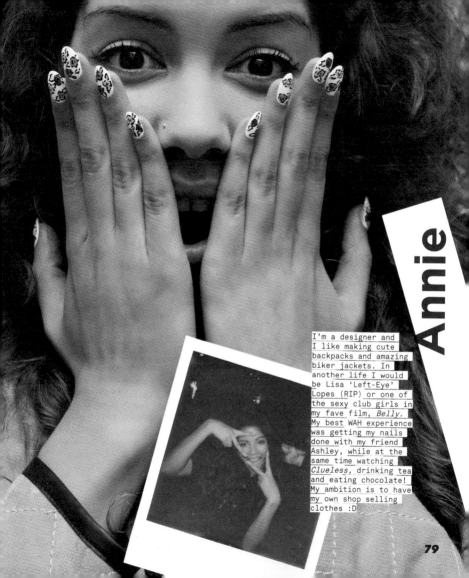

Annie

I'm a designer and I like making cute backpacks and amazing biker jackets. In another life I would be Lisa 'Left-Eye' Lopes (RIP) or one of the sexy club girls in my fave film, *Belly*. My best WAH experience was getting my nails done with my friend Ashley, while at the same time watching *Clueless*, drinking tea and eating chocolate! My ambition is to have my own shop selling clothes :D

Animal prints are the most fun to do on nails and python skin is definitely one for the sophisticated! This design relies on iridescent and shimmery shades to get a real scaly feel. Go for two or three different shades of the same colour and get your sponge at the ready.

STEP 1
Paint your base of light green iridescent polish.

YOU WILL NEED
· light green iridescent polish
· dark green shimmer polish
· black nail-art pen

STEP 2
Paint a little dark green polish onto your sponge and dab a line down the centre of each nail.

PYTHON SKIN

STEP 3
Using your black nail pen draw a loose zig-zag down the nail.

STEP 5
Repeat on the other side of the nail until your whole nail is covered.

STEP 4
Using the zig-zag line as your guide, draw small semi-circle zig-zags or scallops, going smaller as you reach the edge of the nail.

TOP TIP
WORK ON GETTING A SUPER THIN LINE WITH YOUR NAIL-ART PEN. USE IT TOO THICKLY AND IT WILL GO BLOBBY!

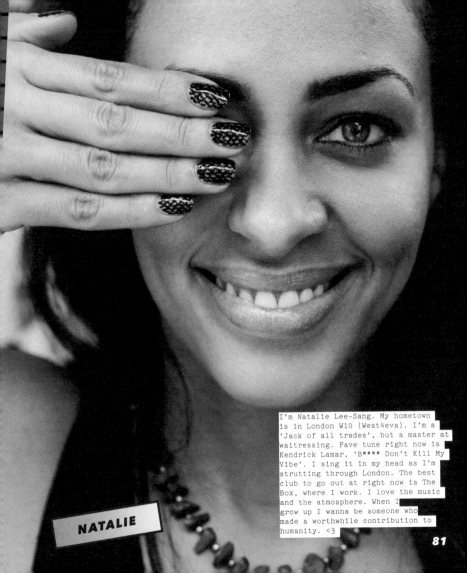

I'm Natalie Lee-Sang. My hometown is in London W10 (West4eva). I'm a 'Jack of all trades', but a master at waitressing. Fave tune right now is Kendrick Lamar, 'B**** Don't Kill My Vibe'. I sing it in my head as I'm strutting through London. The best club to go out at right now is The Box, where I work. I love the music and the atmosphere. When I grow up I wanna be someone who made a worthwhile contribution to humanity. <3

NATALIE

Drippy

One of our original, and favourite, designs! Sometimes inspiration comes from the products themselves and we came up with this design when we were given the most delicious, chocolately nail polish we'd ever seen! We swiftly created an ice-cream drip nail and since then we've changed the colours to create green slime, red blood and pink paint. It's a real hit with our clientele.

YOU WILL NEED >
• pink polish
• black nail-art pen

HOW TO >
Step 1. Paint your nails with the pink base colour. Allow to dry.

Step 2. Using your black nail-art pen, start near the bottom of the nail and paint the outline of a long drip and a mini drip.

Step 3. Continue to paint a long, fat drip in the middle.

Step 4. End the drips with some of smaller in length, making each finger different for a unique effect.

Step 5. Squeeze the nail pen out to fill the drippy area with solid black. You can add some smaller splats off the main one for a cool variation!

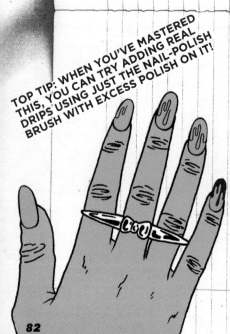

TOP TIP: WHEN YOU'VE MASTERED THIS, YOU CAN TRY ADDING REAL DRIPS USING JUST THE NAIL-POLISH BRUSH WITH EXCESS POLISH ON IT!

82

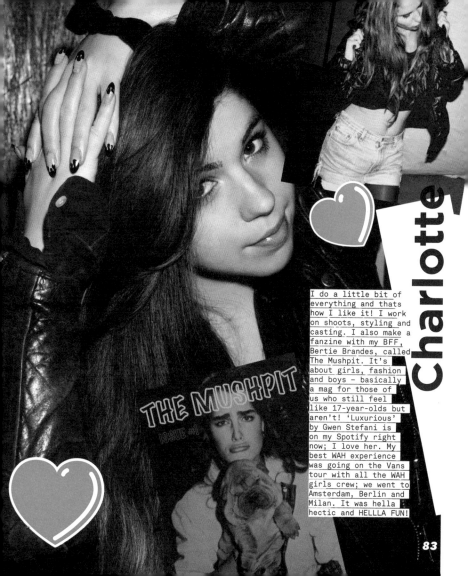

Charlotte

I do a little bit of everything and thats how I like it! I work on shoots, styling and casting. I also make a fanzine with my BFF, Bertie Brandes, called The Mushpit. It's about girls, fashion and boys – basically a mag for those of us who still feel like 17-year-olds but aren't! 'Luxurious' by Gwen Stefani is on my Spotify right now; I love her. My best WAH experience was going on the Vans tour with all the WAH girls crew; we went to Amsterdam, Berlin and Milan. It was hella hectic and HELLLA FUN!

THE MUSHPIT

ISSUE #1

Got something to say? Say it with your nails! There are many types of writing you can do on your nails, but we think script writing is cool as it connects all your nails together to form a message. We did these nails for our friend Ashley William's debut collection at London Fashion Week. She wanted to CELEBRATE so we whipped these up for her. One or two letters per nail works well and it's a good chance to get practising with your nail-art pen.

YOU WILL NEED
· blue polish
· white nail pen

SCRIPT WRITING

STEP 1
On a piece of paper write out your word in joined up writing. Add flourishes to the end of letters to add to the effect.

STEP 2
Using your white nail pen, paint a large, cursive 'C' on your thumb nail. Make sure the end of the letter comes off the nail.

STEP 5
Allow to dry fully before top coating. As the white will be thick, you don't want to ruin your design by dragging your polish through it.

STEP 4
Repeat until you have finished your word 'CELEBRATE' ensure the words starts off the nail and finishes off the nail.

STEP 3
Starting from the edge of the nail draw a lower case 'e' on the left side of the nail and flow it around to an 'l' Make sure the 'l' comes off the nail.

celebrate

TOP TIP
PRACTICE YOUR WORD USING YOUR NAIL PEN ON A PIECE OF PAPER BEFORE STARTING.

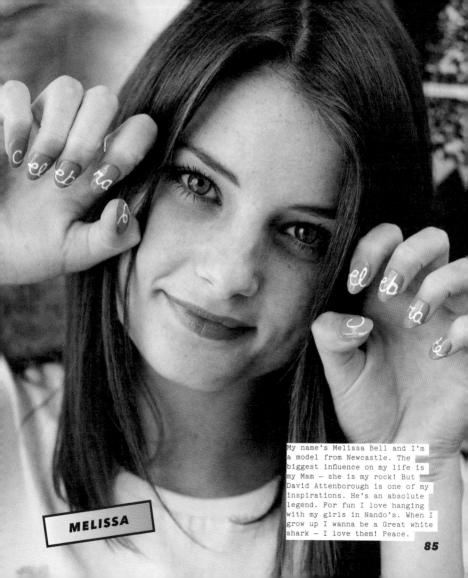

My name's Melissa Bell and I'm a model from Newcastle. The biggest influence on my life is my Mam — she is my rock! But David Attenborough is one of my inspirations. He's an absolute legend. For fun I love hanging with my girls in Nando's. When I grow up I wanna be a Great white shark — I love them! Peace.

MELISSA

85

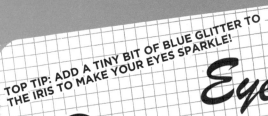

Eyeball

This one's not just for Halloween!
Get gruesome with these bloodshot
eyeballs!

YOU WILL NEED >
- white polish
- blue nail-art pen
- black nail-art pen
- white nail-art pen
- red nail-art pen

HOW TO >
Step 1. Paint your nails with the
white base colour. It can get messy
so don't go too close to your cuticles
and skin. Allow to dry.

Step 2. Using the blue nail-art pen,
draw a circle outline in the centre
of the nail. Next, gently squeeze nail
polish out of the nail-art pen to fill
the circle completely.

Step 3. Add a smaller black circle in the
centre, using the black nail-art pen.

Step 4. Squeeze your white nail pen
until a tiny white ball of polish forms
on the end of the nib. Stop squeezing
and gently touch the ball onto the side
of the black dot. Make sure the nib
itself doesn't touch the nail, just
the ball of polish. This will add a
reflection spot on your eyeball.

Step 5. Take your red nail-art pen
and work inwards from the edge of the
nail to create the blood veins. Make
lightning-bolt and Y-shaped jagged lines
to make them look authentic.

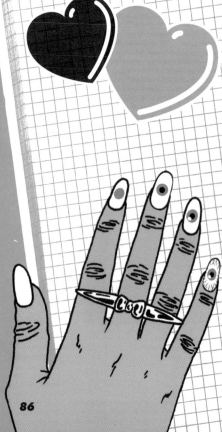

86

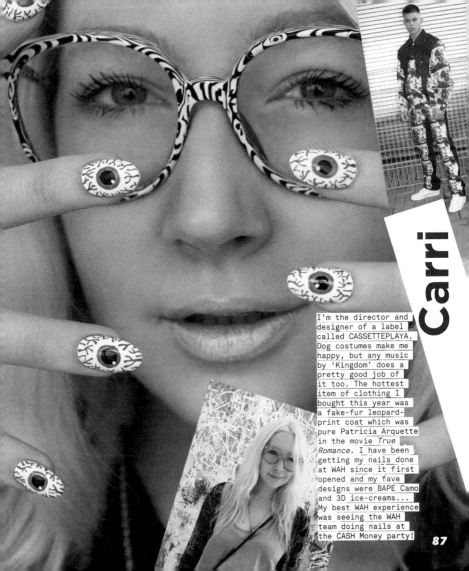

Carri

I'm the director and designer of a label called CASSETTEPLAYA. Dog costumes make me happy, but any music by 'Kingdom' does a pretty good job of it too. The hottest item of clothing I bought this year was a fake-fur leopard-print coat which was pure Patricia Arquette in the movie *True Romance*. I have been getting my nails done at WAH since it first opened and my fave designs were BAPE Camo and 3D ice-creams... My best WAH experience was seeing the WAH team doing nails at the CASH Money party!

87

Cute and preppy, sneaker nails are so simple yet effective. Pick bold primary colours or try a fade underneath for a twist.

THIS IS A GREAT ONE FOR SHORT NAILS!

STEP 1
Paint on your base colours, do every nail different or keep them all the same. It's up to you!

STEP 2
Using a white polish and your striper do an upside down half moon at the bottom of your nail.

YOU WILL NEED
· red polish
· yellow polish
· green polish
· blue polish
· white polish
. black nail-art pen
· black striper

SNEAKER

STEP 5
Using a black striper, paint a smile shape line from one side of your nail to the other (on top of your white half moon), just a little bit up from the bottom of your nail. Don't forget to top coat!

STEP 3
Still using your striper paint on the laces. Start with the line at the top then the two crosses underneath.

STEP 4
Next, use your black pen to dot on your lace holes at the end of each lace line. The black dots should all line up on each side.

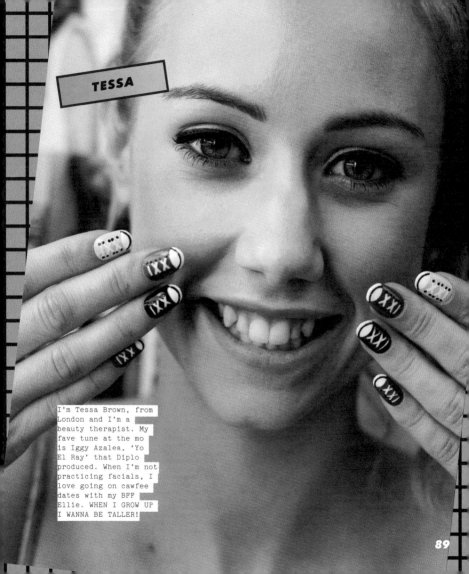

I'm Tessa Brown, from London and I'm a beauty therapist. My fave tune at the mo is Iggy Azalea, 'Yo El Ray' that Diplo produced. When I'm not practicing facials, I love going on cawfee dates with my BFF Ellie. WHEN I GROW UP I WANNA BE TALLER!

TOP TIP: IF YOUR HAND ISN'T STEADY ENOUGH TO
CREATE NEAT LINES, USE BLACK NAIL STRIPING
TAPE TO FINISH OFF YOUR DESIGN.

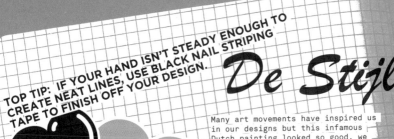

De Stijl

Many art movements have inspired us
in our designs but this infamous
Dutch painting looked so good, we
applied it, literally.

YOU WILL NEED >
- white polish
- red nail striper
- blue nail striper
- yellow nail striper
- black nail-art pen

HOW TO >
Step 1. Paint your nails with the white
base colour. Allow to dry.

Step 2. Using your red striper, draw a
large square outline on the left side of
the nail, that takes up about a third of
the nail area. Fill in the square with red.

Step 3. Take your blue striper and
create a smaller blue triangular shape
at the bottom of the nail that just
touches the red square. Fill in with
blue. Use your yellow striper to create
a small yellow triangle at the tip of
the nail, not quite touching the red
square, and fill in with yellow.

Step 4. Once the colours are dry, use
your black nail-art pen to draw straight
lines between the red, yellow and blue
shapes, so that they are all outined.

Step 5. To finish, add a small black
outline under the yellow triangle and
two small vertical lines under the red
square.

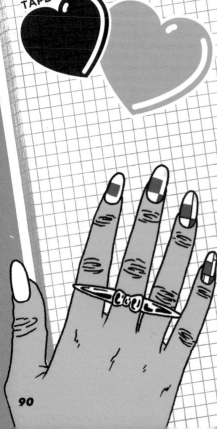

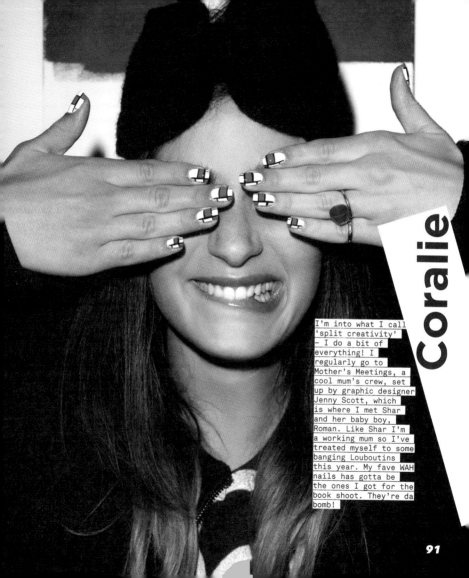

Coralie

I'm into what I call 'split creativity' – I do a bit of everything! I regularly go to Mother's Meetings, a cool mum's crew, set up by graphic designer Jenny Scott, which is where I met Shar and her baby boy, Roman. Like Shar I'm a working mum so I've treated myself to some banging Louboutins this year. My fave WAH nails has gotta be the ones I got for the book shoot. They're da bomb!

For those who don't have an airbrush machine at home, it's still totally possible to create splatter and spray look nails with this easy design. Neon colours look great. Just ensure each layer of colour dries throughly before sponging the second one one.

YOU WILL NEED
· white polish
· yellow polish
· sponge
· clean striper brush
· pink polish
· black polish

SPLATTER

STEP 1
Paint your nail with the white base colour.

STEP 2
Paint a little yellow polish on your sponge and dab a spot on your nail.

STEP 5
Repeat with the black.

STEP 4
Repeat using a pink colour.

STEP 3
Using your clean striper brush, dip into the same yellow polish colour and let the polish gently drip from the sponge spot on your nail.

TOP TIP
START WITH THE LIGHTEST COLOUR FIRST SO THAT YOU WONT HAVE OVERSHADOWING.

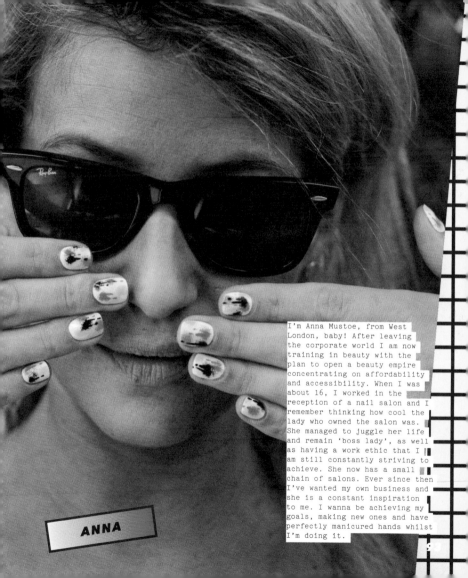

I'm Anna Mustoe, from West
London, baby! After leaving
the corporate world I am now
training in beauty with the
plan to open a beauty empire
concentrating on affordability
and accessibility. When I was
about 16, I worked in the
reception of a nail salon and I
remember thinking how cool the
lady who owned the salon was.
She managed to juggle her life
and remain 'boss lady', as well
as having a work ethic that I
am still constantly striving to
achieve. She now has a small
chain of salons. Ever since then
I've wanted my own business and
she is a constant inspiration
to me. I wanna be achieving my
goals, making new ones and have
perfectly manicured hands whilst
I'm doing it.

ANNA

Graphic Stripe

TOP TIP: IF YOU HAVE SHORT NAILS, YOU COULD EASILY SWITCH THIS DESIGN TO RUN VERTICALLY, WHICH WOULD GIVE THE APPEARANCE OF LENGTHENING YOUR NAIL BED.

Sometimes you just gotta get serious with your nails and stripes are a fail-safe way to do that. We've gone for black, gold and pink, our fave colour combo, but these would look even more sombre and graphic in a monotone.

YOU WILL NEED >
• gold polish
• white polish
• pink nail striper
• black nail striper

HOW TO >
Step 1. Paint your nails alternately with the gold and white base colours. Allow to dry.

Step 2. Using your pink striper, paint a neat straight line across the bottom third of your nail. Fill in to your cuticle area using the tip of your striper brush.

Step 3. In the top third of your nail, repeat using the black striper.

Step 4. Still using the black striper, paint a straight horizontal line in the centre of the nail.

Step 5. Pull out your pink striper again to add a fine pink line just under your black block at the tip of your nail.

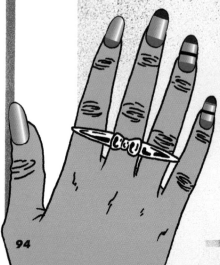

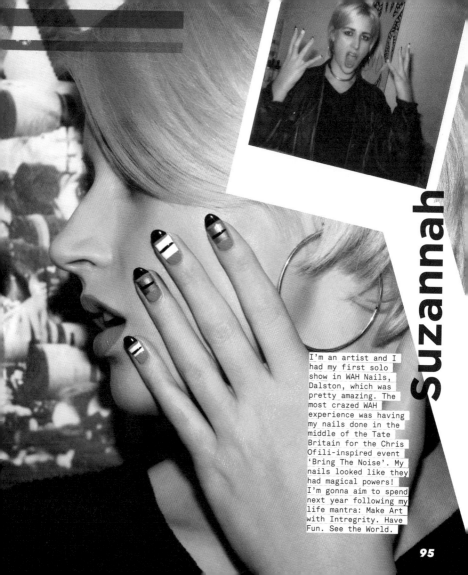

Suzannah

I'm an artist and I had my first solo show in WAH Nails, Dalston, which was pretty amazing. The most crazed WAH experience was having my nails done in the middle of the Tate Britain for the Chris Ofili-inspired event 'Bring The Noise'. My nails looked like they had magical powers! I'm gonna aim to spend next year following my life mantra: Make Art with Intregrity. Have Fun. See the World.

Totally inspired by our fave babes in the film *Clueless*, this tartan design looks great on short, square nails. Like most of our designs, it's a whole lot easier if you have an actual swatch of tartan fabric to replicate. Keep practicising those straight lines!

YOU WILL NEED
· red polish
· white striper
· black nail-art pen
. black striper
· yellow striper

TARTAN

STEP 1
Paint the nails in a base colour of red.

STEP 2
Using a white striper, paint two lines vertically down the nail and two white lines horizontally across the nail.

STEP 3
Where the white stripes cross over, paint four little black squares over them using a nail-art pen.

STEP 4
Continuing with the nail-art pen make little diagonal dashes over the rest of the white stripes.

STEP 5
Using a black striper, paint a line vertically and horizontally to frame the nail. To make it stand out more, follow the same lines again with a yellow striper.

TOP TIP
THIS DESIGNS LOOKS AMAZE WITH THE COLOURS FLIPPED! A YELLOW BASE WITH RED LINES

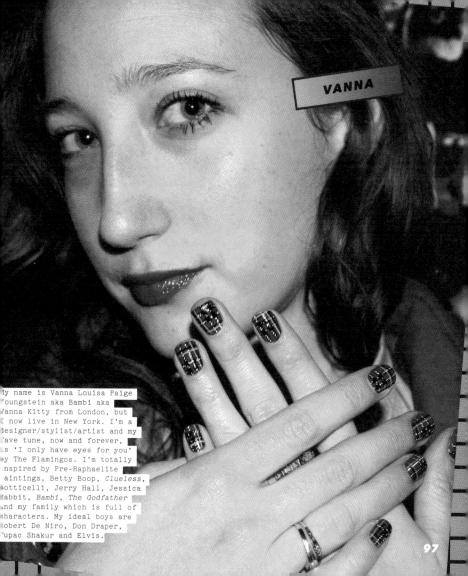

My name is Vanna Louisa Paige Youngstein aka Bambi aka Vanna Kitty from London, but now live in New York. I'm a designer/stylist/artist and my rave tune, now and forever, is 'I only have eyes for you' by The Flamingos. I'm totally inspired by Pre-Raphaelite paintings, Betty Boop, *Clueless*, Botticelli, Jerry Hall, Jessica Rabbit, *Bambi*, *The Godfather* and my family which is full of characters. My ideal boys are Robert De Niro, Don Draper, Tupac Shakur and Elvis.

Lips

Depending on the size and length of the nail, you may be able to get two to three sets of lips on each one. Have a picture of some lips on hand to draw from, to help you create the right shape. You can also experiment with colours – black lips on a pink base look amaze!

YOU WILL NEED >
• pink polish
• red nail striper

HOW TO >
Step 1. Paint your nails with the pink base colour. Allow to dry.

Step 2. Get your red nail-art pen and test the colour quickly on a paper towel. You want to get rid of any air bubbles in the pen.

Step 3. Draw the outline of a set of lips towards the bottom of the nail, at a slight angle.

Step 4. Fill in the lips with the red nail-art pen, leaving a small gap in the middle for the mouth and taking care not to go outside your outline.

Step 5. Repeat this two more times on the nail. Start drawing your second set of lips in the middle of the nail, at an opposing angle to the one at the bottom, and fill them in. Draw your final lips at the tip of the nail at a differing angle again, then fill them in as above.

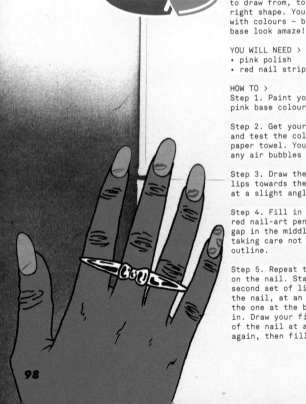

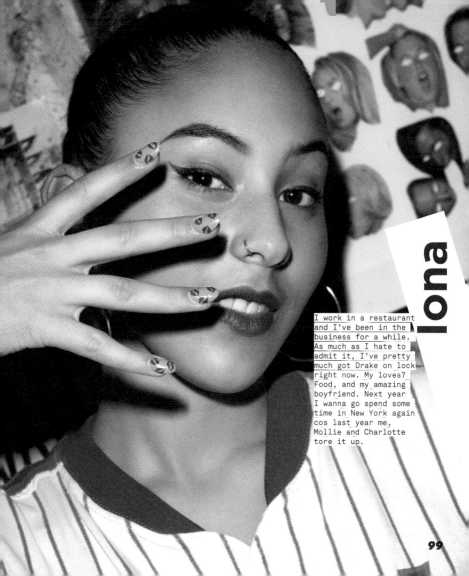

Iona

I work in a restaurant and I've been in the business for a while. As much as I hate to admit it, I've pretty much got Drake on lock right now. My loves? Food, and my amazing boyfriend. Next year I wanna go spend some time in New York again cos last year me, Mollie and Charlotte tore it up.

What we love about this nail design is that it takes the basic elements of an old nail design 'fade away', and with a little flip and a simple change of colours, you can create something totally relevant and new. This design is all about summer festival vibe!

YOU WILL NEED

· white polish
· yellow pastel polish
· pink pastel polish
· turquoise polish
· blue polish
· purple polish
· sponge

TIE-DYE FADE

STEP 1
First paint your nails a white base colour and allow it to dry. This helps the colours you use stay really vibrant and makes them easier to blend.

STEP 2
Then paint the darker of the two colours you're using on one half of the nail.

STEP 3
Using the lighter colour repeat the process on the other side, slightly Overlapping the first colour.

STEP 4
Then using a sponge dab the lighter colour you've used, up the middle of the nail, overlapping the darker colour. Keep doing this to build up the gradient effect of the two colours blending.

STEP 5
Repeat the process on each nail using your different colours.

TOP TIP
YOU CAN ALSO USE A PALETTE AND BLEND THE TWO COLOURS BEFORE APPLYING TO THE NAIL, JUST MIX THE COLOURS TOGETHER AND USE THE SPONGE TO DAB ON THE MIDDLE OF THE NAIL.

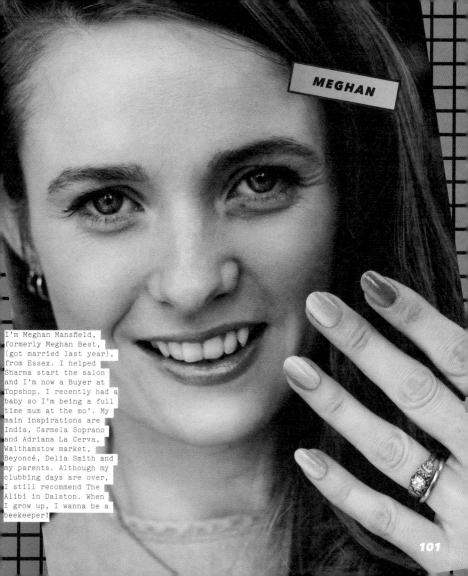

MEGHAN

I'm Meghan Mansfield,
formerly Meghan Best,
(got married last year),
from Essex. I helped
Sharma start the salon
and I'm now a Buyer at
Topshop. I recently had a
baby so I'm being a full
time mum at the mo'. My
main inspirations are
India, Carmela Soprano
and Adriana La Cerva,
Walthamstow market,
Beyoncé, Delia Smith and
my parents. Although my
clubbing days are over,
I still recommend The
Alibi in Dalston. When
I grow up, I wanna be a
beekeeper!

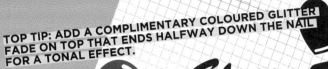

TOP TIP: ADD A COMPLIMENTARY COLOURED GLITTER FADE ON TOP THAT ENDS HALFWAY DOWN THE NAIL FOR A TONAL EFFECT.

Glitter Fade

Sometimes you just need a bit of sparkle to make life okay. Try this quick and easy design for an instant update to plain nails.

YOU WILL NEED >
• black polish
• gold glitter polish

HOW TO >
1. Paint your nails with the black base colour. Allow to dry.

2. Load up your glitter polish brush and blob the glitter along the tip of the nail.

3. Wipe the polish brush clean on the rim of the bottle, so it's almost dry, and then starting from the centre, drag the polish down towards the cuticle.

4. Continue with the left-side of the nail, dragging the glitter polish from the tip, down towards the cuticle with the dry brush, to create the fade.

5. Drag right edge down to the cuticle and fill in any gaps with tiny amounts of glitter.

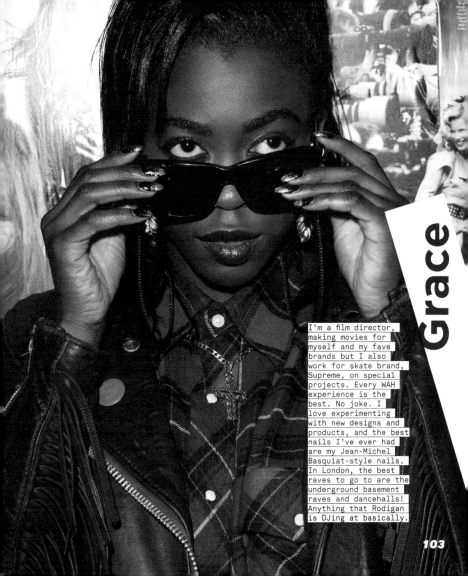

Grace

I'm a film director,
making movies for
myself and my fave
brands but I also
work for skate brand,
Supreme, on special
projects. Every WAH
experience is the
best. No joke. I
love experimenting
with new designs and
products, and the best
nails I've ever had
are my Jean-Michel
Basquiat-style nails.
In London, the best
raves to go to are the
underground basement
raves and dancehalls!
Anything that Rodigan
is DJing at basically.

We made this design pretty early on in the salon when we became obsessed with tie-dyeing all of our clothes (we were gonna start a brand called Tie Or Dye! Lol) and wanted nails to match! Try this with our IMMERGE collection. If want to add black into your design it looks amazing and inky.

STEP 1
Work on one nail at a time and begin by blobbing the yellow nail varnish in a big strip across the base nail.

STEP 2
Leaving a gap in the middle of your nail, dab a thick strip of yellow polish on the tip of the nail.

YOU WILL NEED
· yellow polish
· orange polish
· cocktail stick

TIE-DYE SWIRL

STEP 5
Add more colour if you feel its uneven or lacking and then wait at least ten minutes before applying the topcoat as the nail polish will be thick.

STEP 4
Using a cocktail or cuticle stick and gently drag the colours into each other in a swirling pattern.

STEP 3
Working quickly, with your orange polish, blob a large strip across the middle of the nail. overlap with the yellow and you start to see the colours mix.

TOP TIP
IF YOU FIND YOU ARE SCRATCHING THE POLISH ALL THE WAY TO THE BASE OF THE NAIL, YOU CAN DO A BASE OF YELLOW AND LET IT DRY.

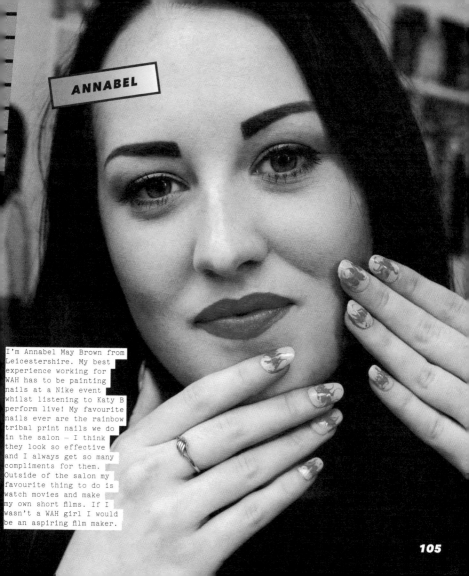

I'm Annabel May Brown from Leicestershire. My best experience working for WAH has to be painting nails at a Nike event whilst listening to Katy B perform live! My favourite nails ever are the rainbow tribal print nails we do in the salon — I think they look so effective and I always get so many compliments for them. Outside of the salon my favourite thing to do is watch movies and make my own short films. If I wasn't a WAH girl I would be an aspiring film maker.

Marble

TOP TIP: THIS DESIGN LOOKS BEST WITH BLACK, WHITE AND ANY OTHER COLOUR. DON'T DRAG MORE THAN THREE LINES IN EITHER DIRECTION OR IT WILL JUST LOOK LIKE A MESS!

Do one nail at a time on this one, as you want your polish to be wet when you start to create the marble effect.

YOU WILL NEED >
- beige polish
- white polish
- black polish
- cocktail stick

HOW TO >

Step 1. Paint your nails with the beige base colour. Allow to dry.

Step 2. Take your white nail polish and use the brush to add three blobs of polish to the nail.

Step 3. Add a couple of black polish blobs to the nail. You don't have to be really precise with this part, as marble nails look best when they aren't all uniform.

Step 4. Drag a cocktail stick vertically across the nail to create three marbled lines. Be careful not to press too hard, as your don't want to drag the base colour off the nail bed.

Step 5. Now use the cocktail stick to create three horizontal lines. Have fun with this design, it's not about being exact on this one.

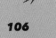

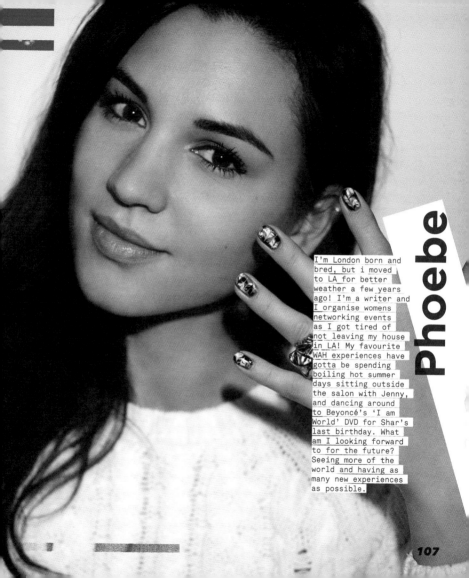

Phoebe

I'm London born and bred, but i moved to LA for better weather a few years ago! I'm a writer and I organise womens networking events as I got tired of not leaving my house in LA! My favourite WAH experiences have gotta be spending boiling hot summer days sitting outside the salon with Jenny, and dancing around to Beyoncé's 'I am World' DVD for Shar's last birthday. What am I looking forward to for the future? Seeing more of the world and having as many new experiences as possible.

There is so much to be done with black and white polish and a great monochrome design is woven nails. It may look detailed but once you get a rhythm you can cover each nail in a minute or so, making this a quick and easy design.

YOU WILL NEED
· white polish
· black nail pen

STEP 1
Paint your nails in your white base colour.

STEP 2
Starting in the centre of the nail draw three lines vertically using a nail-art pen.

WOVEN

STEP 5
Allow to dry fully before painting your topcoat.

STEP 4
Repeat this column in the same way and fill the nail in the same way with horizontal next to vertical.

STEP 3
Below this, draw three lines horizontally, the same length as the three lines above are wide.

TOP TIP
TAKE IT TO THE NEXT LEVEL BY DOING TWO DIFFERENT COLOURED WEAVES, SO ALL HORIZONTAL LINES ARE ONE COLOUR AND ALL VERTICAL LINES ARE A SECOND COLOUR.

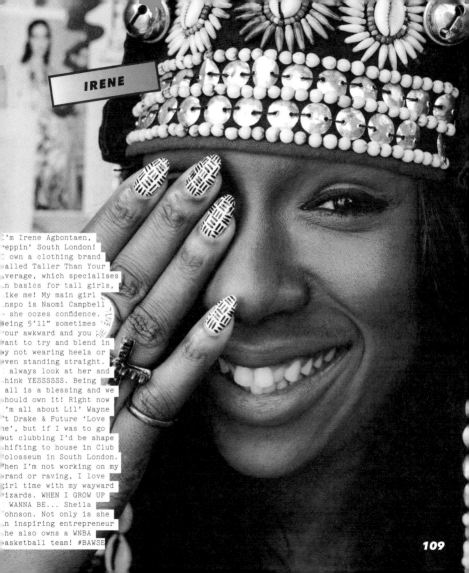

I'm Irene Agbontaen, reppin' South London! I own a clothing brand called Taller Than Your Average, which specialises in basics for tall girls, like me! My main girl inspo is Naomi Campbell – she oozes confidence. Being 5'11" sometimes your awkward and you want to try and blend in by not wearing heels or even standing straight. I always look at her and think YESSSSSS. Being tall is a blessing and we should own it! Right now I'm all about Lil' Wayne ft Drake & Future 'Love Me', but if I was to go out clubbing I'd be shape shifting to house in Club Colosseum in South London. When I'm not working on my brand or raving, I love girl time with my wayward lizards. WHEN I GROW UP I WANNA BE... Sheila Johnson. Not only is she an inspiring entrepreneur she also owns a WNBA basketball team! #BAWSE

109

Rhinestone Rain

Make it rain jewels, not money, with these crystal-studded nail stars! Swarovski crystals work best with this design. Choose a dark stone, a light stone, and a white stone for a cool sparkle effect.

YOU WILL NEED >
• pink polish
• glitter polish
• nail glue
• cocktail stick
• large, medium and small rhinestones or Swarovski crystals
• top coat

HOW TO >
Step 1. Paint your nails with the pink base colour. Allow to dry, then add a light coat of glitter, fading halfway down the nail.

Step 2. Dab three drops of nail glue onto the nail. Dip your cocktail stick in some top coat, use it to pick up a large gem, then press it in place onto the nail. Follow with two more gems. The glue will take a few seconds to dry, so try not to touch them until they're secure.

Step 3. Using the same method, stick on your medium-sized rhinestones, interspersing them amongst the larger gems.

Step 4. Fill in any gaps with the small rhinestones. These little ones can be a bit fiddly to apply, but practice makes perfect!

Step 5. Add more small rhinestones trickling down the nail to get the full Rhinestone Rain effect!

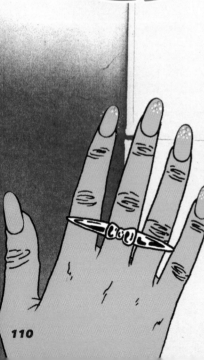

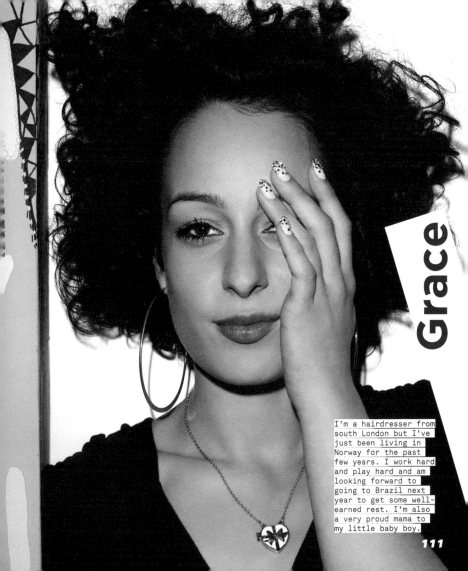

Grace

I'm a hairdresser from south London but I've just been living in Norway for the past few years. I work hard and play hard and am looking forward to going to Brazil next year to get some well-earned rest. I'm also a very proud mama to my little baby boy.

Girls are complex. One minute you love pink hair, the next you hate it; one day you wanna be an artist, the next day you wanna be a financier. That's why we love the ying and yang design — the idea of two completely opposite forces, complementing each other and forming a whole. Can't decide if you want black or white nails? No worries! Have both colours with this nail design.

YOU WILL NEED
· white polish
· black striper
· black polish
· black nail-art pen
· white nail-art pen

YING YANG

STEP 1
Paint all your nails in your white base colour.

STEP 2
Using your black striper draw the ying yang curve. Best way to get the perfect curve is to draw an 'S' shape!

STEP 3
Fill in one side of your 'S' with the black keeping the neatest line on the white side.

STEP 4
Using your black pen draw a circle on the white side and fill in.

STEP 5
Using your white nail-art pen, draw a circle on the black side and fill in.

TOP TIP
TAKE IT TO THE NEXT LEVEL ONCE YOUVE MASTERED THIS DESIGN DO A CUTE MINI VERSION WITH A BRIGHT NEON BASE!

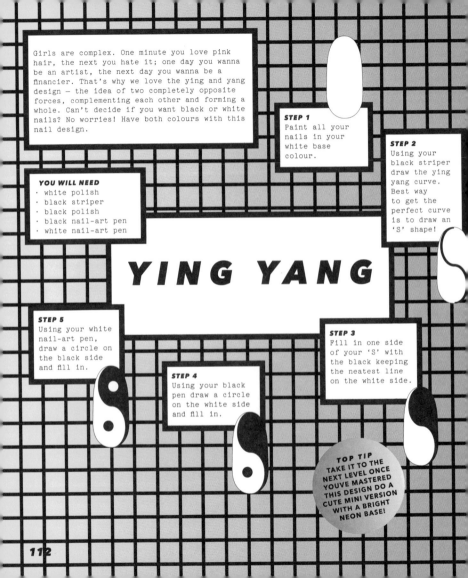

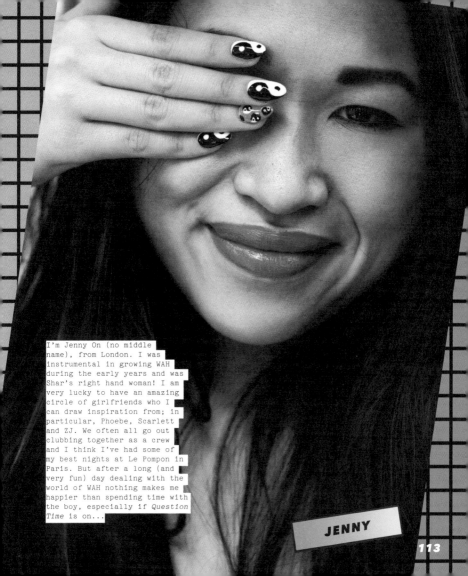

I'm Jenny On (no middle name), from London. I was instrumental in growing WAH during the early years and was Shar's right hand woman! I am very lucky to have an amazing circle of girlfriends who I can draw inspiration from; in particular, Phoebe, Scarlett and ZJ. We often all go out clubbing together as a crew and I think I've had some of my best nights at Le Pompon in Paris. But after a long (and very fun) day dealing with the world of WAH nothing makes me happier than spending time with the boy, especially if *Question Time* is on...

JENNY

Double Studs

Gold on your nails will always look impressive, and these studs are surprisingly easy to apply! Find nail studs at your local craft store for an instant party look.

YOU WILL NEED >
• black polish
• gold studs
• cocktail stick
• top coat

HOW TO >
Step 1. Paint your nails with the black base colour. Allow to dry.

Step 2. Place a few dabs of the top coat near the base of the nail.

Step 3. Using the cocktail stick, gently touch the top coat blob on the nail – you want just a small amount on the end of your stick. Then quickly use the wet cocktail stick to pick up a stud and place two at the base of the nail on the top coat blob.

Step 4. Working away from the base, continue to place dabs of top coat and studs until the nail is full.

Step 5. Go and brush your shoulders off!

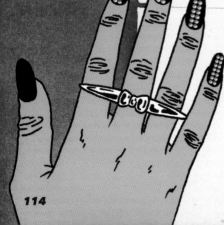

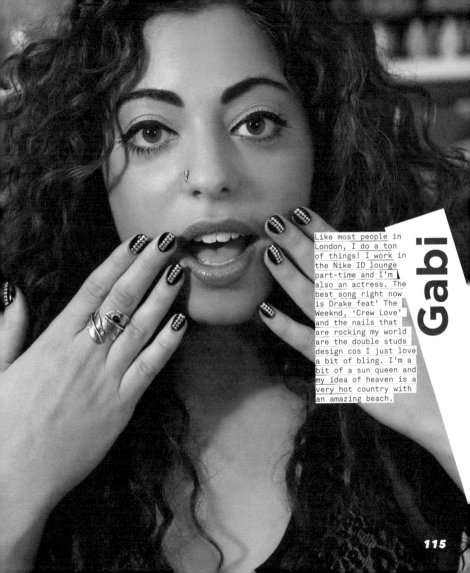

Like most people in London, I do a ton of things! I work in the Nike ID lounge part-time and I'm also an actress. The best song right now is Drake feat' The Weeknd, 'Crew Love' and the nails that are rocking my world are the double studs design cos I just love a bit of bling. I'm a bit of a sun queen and my idea of heaven is a very hot country with an amazing beach.

Gabi

These tropical zig-zags look amazing with bright backgrounds or a coloured fade. Whether you use the striper or the nail pen is totally up to you! Figure out what tool you can manage the best, but if it is your striper, ensure that you have no loose bristle or they'll ruin your perfect lines.

STEP 1
Paint your base colour on all your nails and using your highlight colour, paint onto your sponge and dab a few spots over the nail.

STEP 2
Start in the centre of the nail and paint one zig-zag in the middle of the nail to start you off.

ZIG-ZAG

STEP 5
Repeat zig-zag lines all the way to the tip of your nail.

STEP 3
Complete the zig-zag to the left and right to create one long zig-zag going across centre of the nail.

STEP 4
Using your first line as a guide, repeat zig-zag lines towards the base of your nails.

TOP TIP
MAKE YOUR ZIG-ZAG LINES GET SMALLER AS THEY REACH THE BASE AND TIP OF THE NAIL FOR AN OPTICAL ILLUSION EFFECT!

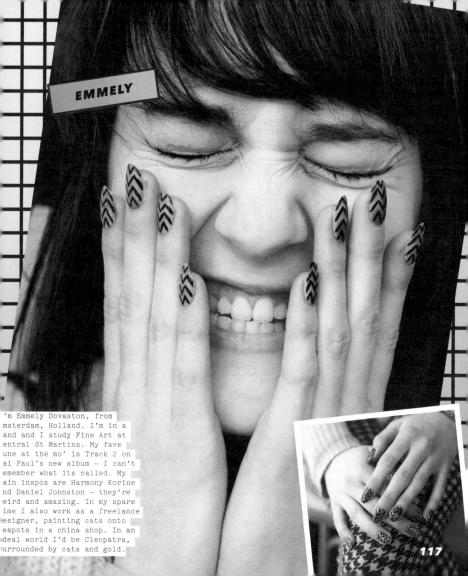

'm Emmely Dovaston, from
msterdam, Holland. I'm in a
and and I study Fine Art at
entral St Martins. My fave
une at the mo' is Track 2 on
ai Paul's new album — I can't
emember what its called. My
ain inspos are Harmony Korine
nd Daniel Johnston — they're
eird and amazing. In my spare
ime I also work as a freelance
esigner, painting cats onto
eapots in a china shop. In an
deal world I'd be Cleopatra,
urrounded by cats and gold.

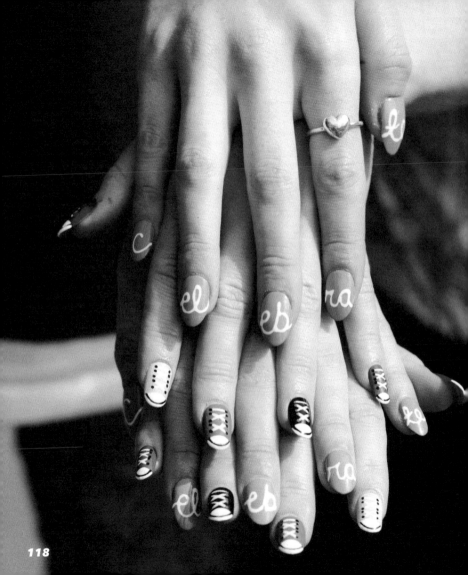

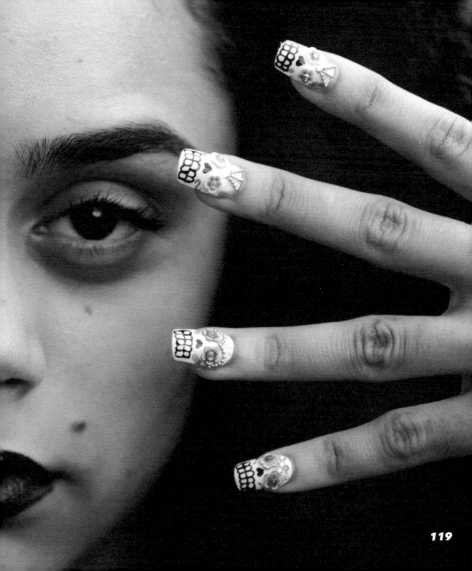

Design your own...

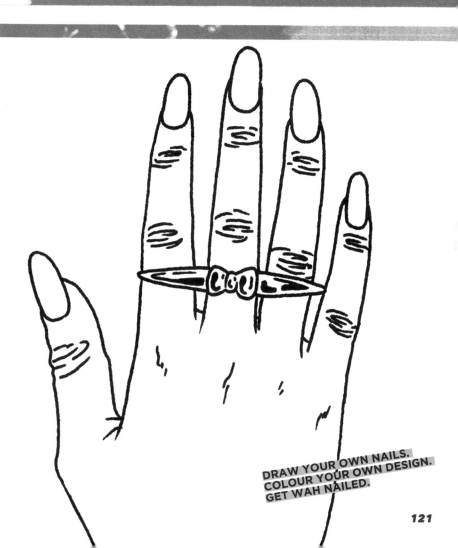

DRAW YOUR OWN NAILS.
COLOUR YOUR OWN DESIGN.
GET WAH NAILED.

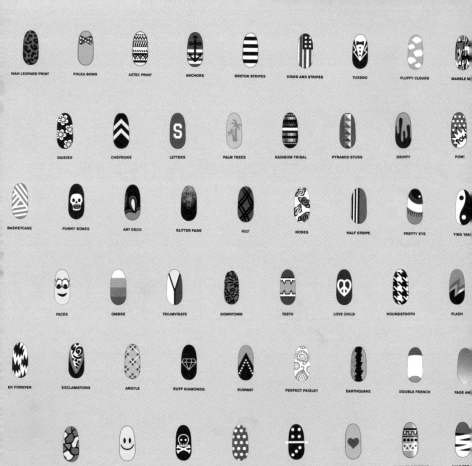

WAH LEOPARD PRINT

POLKA BOWS

AZTEC PRINT

ANCHORS

BRETON STRIPES

STARS AND STRIPES

TUXEDO

FLUFFY CLOUDS

MARBLE M

DAISIES

CHEVRONS

LETTERS

PALM TREES

RAINBOW TRIBAL

PYRAMID STUDS

DRIPPY

POW!

BASKETCASE

FUNNY BONES

ART DECO

GLITTER FADE

KILT

ROSES

HALF STRIPE

PRETTY EYE

YING YAN

FACES

OMBRE

TRIUMVIRATE

DOWNTOWN

TEETH

LOVE CHILD

HOUNDSTOOTH

FLASH

EK FOREVER

EXCLAMATIONS

ARGYLE

RUFF DIAMONDS

RUNWAY

PERFECT PAISLEY

EARTHQUAKE

DOUBLE FRENCH

FADE AW

STAINED GLASS NAILS

DON'T WORRY BE HAPPY

SKULL + CROSS BONES

POLKA DOTS

DOMINO

ONE LOVE

STUDDED EGYPTIAN

HALF ZEB

122

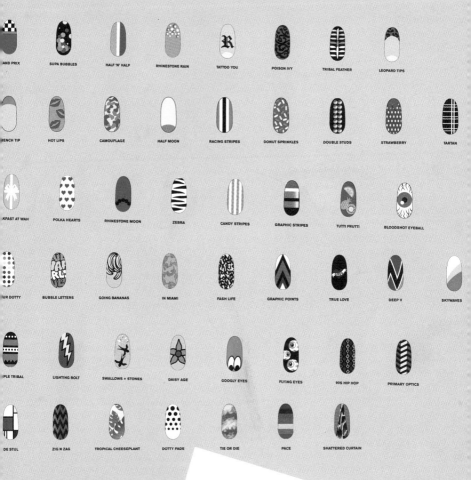

AND PRIX · SUPA BUBBLES · HALF 'N' HALF · RHINESTONE RAIN · TATTOO YOU · POISON IVY · TRIBAL FEATHER · LEOPARD TIPS

FRENCH TIP · HOT LIPS · CAMOUFLAGE · HALF MOON · RACING STRIPES · DONUT SPRINKLES · DOUBLE STUDS · STRAWBERRY · TARTAN

KFAST AT WAH · POLKA HEARTS · RHINESTONE MOON · ZEBRA · CANDY STRIPES · GRAPHIC STRIPES · TUTTI FRUTTI · BLOODSHOT EYEBALL

UR DOTTY · BUBBLE LETTERS · GOING BANANAS · IN MIAMI · FASH LIFE · GRAPHIC POINTS · TRUE LOVE · DEEP V · SKYWAVES

PLE TRIBAL · LIGHTING BOLT · SWALLOWS + STONES · DAISY AGE · GOOGLY EYES · FLYING EYES · 90S HIP HOP · PRIMARY OPTICS

DE STIJL · ZIG N ZAG · TROPICAL CHEESEPLANT · DOTTY FADE · TIE OR DIE · PACE · SHATTERED CURTAIN

The Wah Nails 100

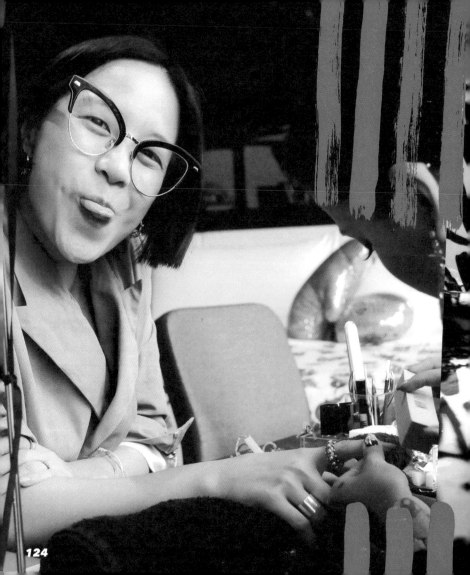

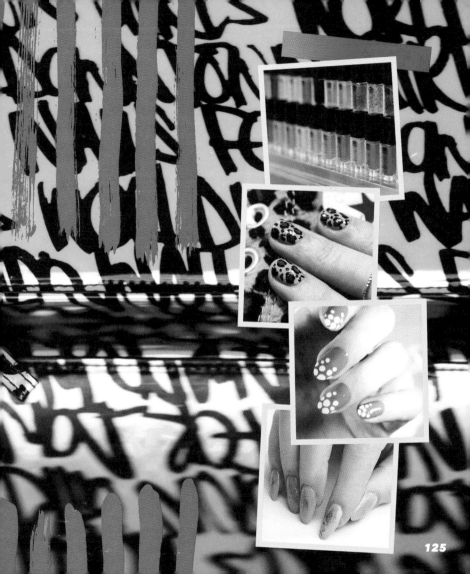

125

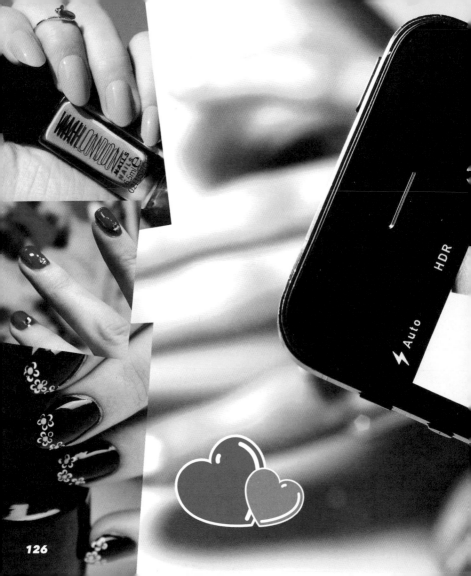

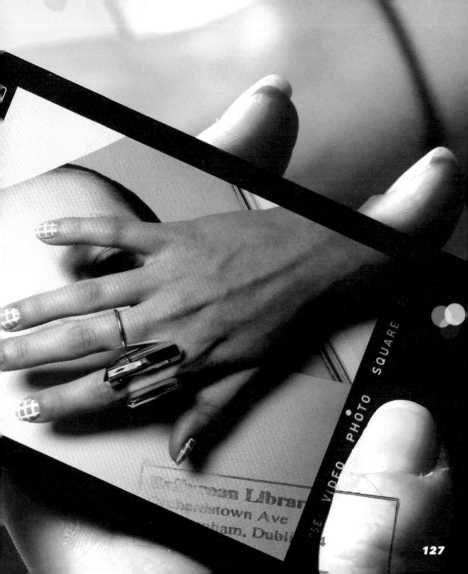

Nails Forever by Sharmadean Reid

First published in 2012 as The WAH Nails Book of Nail Art and in 2013 as The WAH Nails Book of Downtown Girls.
This combined edition published in 2015 by Hardie Grant Books

Hardie Grant Books (UK)
5th & 6th Floors
52-54 Southwark Street
London SE1 1UN
www.hardiegrant.co.uk

Hardie Grant Books (Australia)
Ground Floor, Building 1
658 Church Street
Melbourne, VIC 3121
www.hardiegrant.com.au

British Library Cataloguing-in-Publication Data. A catalogue record for this book is available from the British Library.

ISBN: 978-1-78488-019-4

Publisher: Kate Pollard
Senior Editor: Kajal Mistry
Cover and Art Direction: Sharmadean Reid
Art Direction on pages 6, 7, 16, 17, 20, 21, 23, 24, 28, 29, 32, 33, 36, 37, 40, 41, 44, 45, 48, 49, 52, 53, 56, 57, 60, 61, 64, 64, 70, 71, 74, 75, 78,
79, 82, 83, 86, 87, 90, 91, 94, 95, 98, 99, 102, 103, 106, 107, 110, 111, 114, 115, 120, 121, 122, 123: Rob Meyers for RBPMstudio
Design assistance on cover and on pages 1, 2, 3, 4, 5, 8, 10, 11, 14, 124, 125, 126, 127: Ami Smithson
Design on pages 9, 12, 13, 15, 18, 19, 22, 23, 26, 27, 30, 31, 34, 35, 38, 39, 42, 43, 46, 47, 50, 51, 54, 55, 60, 61, 64, 65, 70, 71, 74, 75, 78, 79,
84, 85, 88, 89, 92, 93, 96, 97, 100, 101, 104, 105, 108, 109, 112, 113, 116, 117:
The New Worlds Projects
Design Assistance on pages 9, 12, 13, 15, 18, 19, 22, 23, 26, 27, 30, 31, 34, 35, 38, 39, 42, 43, 46, 47, 50, 51, 54, 55, 60, 61, 64, 65, 70, 71, 74,
75, 78, 79, 84, 85, 88, 89, 92, 93, 96, 97, 100, 101, 104, 105, 108, 109, 112, 113, 116, 117: Ellie Harry
Retoucher: Steve Crozier
Proofreader: Rose Gardener, Charlotte Roberts

Nails by: Kim Gorse-Macias, Simona Davidikova, Ellie Harry, Poppie Sharman, Julie On, Jessica Thompson, Izzy Bellamy, Kat, Fitzakerly,
Louie-Marie Ebanks, Sharmadean Reid, Georgia Hart, Annabel Brown

Photographs on pages 21, 45, 49, 54, 61, 79, 87, 95 and 115 © Grace Ladoja
Photograph on page 6 © Jordan Stokes
Photographs on pages 17, 24, 25, 33, 37, 41, 65, 71, 75, 83, 91, 99, 103, 107 and 111 © Alex Sainsbury
Polaroid and real film photographs on pages 21, 17, 49, 53, 57, 61, 79, 87 and 95 © Carl Esse
WAH 100 nails illustratrations © Cath Grossider
All other illustrations throughout © Jiro Bevis

Photographs © Robinson Barbosa and Jeff Hahn
Additional Photographs © Simon Hurlstone Archer, Finchittida Finch, Ellie Harry, Bella Howard, Sam Bayliss-Ibram, Erika Maiyagiwa,
Amelia Sechman, Poppie Sharman, Sunny Shokrae, Sharmadean Reid, Charlotte Roberts.

Every attempt has been made to contact the copyright holders. The publishers would like to be contacted by any photographers who have not
been attributed.

Colour Reproduction by p2d and MDP
Printed and bound in China by 1010

10 9 8 7 6 5 4 3 2 1